CONFESSIONS

OF A

Weight Loss Counselor

by

X485

ISBN: 978-1-54390-490-1 (print)
ISBN: 978-1-54390-491-8 (ebook)

TABLE OF CONTENTS

PROLOGUE:

First of all, thank you for buying this book. I can use the money. Is it tacky to begin a prologue this way? Perhaps, but I've been told I lack tact before. So I'll soften it. I'm deeply grateful for your purchase of this book. Even if I didn't need the money, I couldn't be more sincere.

It'd be a wise guess on my part that you have an interest in weight loss. Why else would you have a need for this book? Need this book? Yes, I think you do need it. At least, it's likely. What makes me propose this? One, if you live in America, the odds are simply there. Reports vary, but are grim. Up to 70% of us are overweight. 40% are expected to be beyond overweight and upgraded to obese in the near future. You live in the US; you probably need to lose weight. Two, you're on a computer. As an exclusively online product, I know you attained this book via the internet. How do I link that to being overweight? I confess a bit of literary exaggeration here. Technology baffles me. Yea, yea, it's revolutionized the world and all that. But, it's also made us less active and less willing to come together in physical spaces to revel in the unique power only human contact offers. I do believe we've suffered for that - especially regarding weight management. Three, X485, my professional handle, intrigued you. X = former. 485 is my top weight. It's been off since 2000. I'll never be that person again. It became my life's calling ever since to reach out to anyone willing to be helped. Much like when people enter occupations such as social work, the clergy, special needs education, working with the aged and infirm. You feel called to do it. I've adhered to that call ever since I 'crossed over' and chose a healthy, sane life. Consider this my arm extending to you now.

Throughout this book, you'll read the unfinished work (yes, it is unfinished. I doubt the need will be completely fulfilled in my lifetime) in sections. First will be my life story before, during and since my most recent weight loss. Please notice I did not state this in the absolute. I'm not cured. The work isn't over. It's just a progress report. However, I DO need you to know what I've been through, so my credibility is firmly established in your mind.

Next, you'll be introduced to 40 profiles of people I've dealt with. You'll relate to some, others will have shared identifiable parts, others will read as foreign to you. None are without merit. Plus, lessons to be learned to apply to your own life accompany each, as well.

Next, if I'm successful with you and you feel ready to take your life back, I have a section called The Plan. I'm particularly proud of this section. It gives you some realistic, commonly felt experiences at certain time intervals and how to manage them better. The beginning is so important. Pilot lights are lit, but vulnerable unless they're carefully built upon. These ideas keep fires ignited.

Next, we speculate on why we over consume. Not being a sociologist, I confess my observations here are almost solely taken from my clients and my own life. With over 16 years and 50000+ test cases there have been common threads. I wish to preview my final section, Invitation to Respond, here. I want your additional input. My personal knowledge and research and my 'test bunnies' are all thorough, but never complete. Until I've spoken to every person on the planet, I'll always welcome more. Feel free to offer.

Next, we'll go to the kitchen for some recipes. What Diet Book is without them? You'll find mine unconventional, but I hope useful. They're primary function is not to win contests, impress anyone on the Food Network, or to be called 'amazing', 'better than my mother made' or 'beyond decadently delicious'. They're good, some are very good. Their main purpose is they'll keep you thin and not hungry. A cookbook with that vantage point I've found lacking to suit me. Here, too, I'd love more ideas.

Next, I take you on a trip to the store. I'll strain myself to pat my own back here. Who needs to be given advice on a trip to the store? Many people do! The supermarket in the typical US town needs navigation guidance. Not the usual tour that's generally available, but a dissemination of the entire place in search of the best treasures. I've only taken a few select people to the store and personally, aisle by aisle, guided them. Those few have all called it one of the most valuable experiences they'd had in the battle. It took me years to refine my shopping. I offer some highlights to you.

Finally, an Invitation to Respond. What did you think about a specific profile? How did it compare to you? Which recipes were helpful? I ask for your constructive criticism, confirmation on what you found valuable. I'm grateful for all your two cents.

X485'S STORY:

I'm told I was born hungry, bigger than average from the start. I'm told I was taken to the doctor due to my endless crying and my parents were told to put me on semi solids very early as I was ravenous. First bite, I stop crying and open up my mouth wide for more. Some things never change. Fast forward 50+ years and it's still there: The lure, the obsession. Food, food, food - we need it to survive. But I've had my entire life dictated by it. My mother, obese in my youngest years, was a fantastic cook who thought baking from pre made mixes was sacrilege. Was this a blessing or a curse? Not too sure. Meals were events for me. Both, the home made ones and the processed ones. I craved both, particularly sugar. My, oh, my - sugar. I've been addicted as far as my memory allows and still battle it. Our refrigerator had a freezer on the bottom and I recall getting ice cream out of there: pressing the pedal, pulling off the lid, plunging my fingers into the cold, sweet, gooey stuff. Trying to be quiet and not get caught. As though my finger marks wouldn't get noticed. I'd learn better techniques as I got older. My appetite was endless. I could eat 3 scoops of ice cream by age 6 and often did. There was never enough cereal, peanut butter, chocolate, pie, pasta, French fries, pork chops, cookies, coke, candy bars, pizza, doughnuts - you name it -to fill me up. Food was paradise.

Now, as an adult looking back, how much blame do my parents take for this? I'm torn. My love for them wants to pull my punches here, but the truth forces me to reconsider. As I said, my mother had a life long struggle with her own weight. During my earliest years, she was at her heaviest. Food was the focal point of her life and she did transfer that to me. My father remained on the sidelines about food for the most part. He loved his wife's cooking and ate with gusto, by all means. But, it never quite seemed to overtake him. Don't know why. But, the two of them loved me dearly, this I know. But, the two of them also allowed me too much leeway in this area and I must hold them initially accountable for my overeating at this stage. I do not hold small children entirely answerable for all their behaviors. So, I cannot expect it of me, either. If I'd been reigned in some, would my weight have not been the problem it became? I'll never know. Is there a time when you must accept responsibility for your own actions despite how you were raised? Absolutely! But, my start on this road was, indeed, at my mother and father's hands.

I've heard people say there were raised to 'clean their plates'. Also, that they couldn't go out and play until they finished their dinner. This is like someone telling a bird what a fish does under water. It's so utterly unlike your own experience, it's difficult to comprehend. 'Clean my plate' - HA! I ate so fast and furiously, the only comments I recall were more in the 'slow down!', 'no one's gonna take it away from you' and 'come up for air!' variety. I struggle with the impulse to wolf down my food to this day. A habit I've not overcome. As for the 'I can't go out and play until I finished my dinner' comment - an empty threat for me. I didn't particularly care for the company of other kids. On my first day of school, I got on the bus and there was one other girl, Christie, on there. She looked at me and said, 'Fatso!' It would never end - the entire time I was in school even up and into college.

We dined out frequently and that was a joy. The Sizzler's steaks, potatoes, Texas toast, salads with 1,000 island dressing, many refills of soda pop and dessert - ALWAYS dessert - afterwards. I left most restaurants so full I'd want to unbutton my pants. That was the idea, right?

Las Vegas' most famous dining style is the buffet: glorious, glorious bounty—the buffet. All you can eat. Are you kidding me? All I can eat? Let's DO this! Many Sundays after church, it was buffet and I was delighted. My top problem - having to eat all I wanted with no interruptions. This not-so-little- piggy wanted his meals eaten in big bites and fast. Conversation was not a top priority, chewing, either. Keeping my mouth closed while chewing, in particular. The next bite was usually ready to put in my mouth the second the last bite was being swallowed. UMMM! Manners were a cumbersome issue. Far too restrictive having to cut meat, wipe my mouth, not slurp.... I am not proud of any of this. I am laying out the reality for you, the reader. But I digress, back to buffets. My mother's 1 ever restriction put on my eating came as an 'only one dessert a day' rule. ONE! No way! So, I had to go to the dessert table and shove them in right then and there. Brilliant! Brownie squares inhaled. Pumpkin pie squares went down fast and easy, too. I'd bring one back to the table alter I'd polished off 4 or so.

Food disappeared quickly in my house. I got yelled at often when I'd hear, "I just bought these 3 days ago, get in here!" I'd trudge into the kitchen to answer for 1/2 of the jar of peanut butter being gone, or a row of cookies, a box of cereal or any other delectable thing that I'd snuck at all hours of all days. I'd make excuses that were ridiculous and not believable. To my surprise, one aversion therapy trick worked on me. I was very fond of Fig Newtons and plowed through them like crazy. My mother told me the small seeds were bug heads. I believed her. Their crunchy nature and how small they were all seemed possible to this 8-year-old. It put me off them for many years. MAN, I wish that'd worked more often!

School was not a place of comfort - physically or emotionally. I was very tall for my age and fat, too. Kids made fun of me from the start. "Did you flunk?" was a common question. I was too big to fit in the desks and one from the next grade up had to be brought in for me in 1st, 2nd and 3rd grade. It was horrible being this out of the ordinary: all the desks neatly in a row and then mine. I hated it. In 4th grade, we had wider desks and I spent the whole year sitting sideways, but I was glad to not require a special desk for the first time. So what if I had to twist my neck to see the teacher. Gasp - 5th grade: it was back to the chair attached style desks. No way! I'd learned to protect myself a bit by then. I squeezed myself into a regular sized desk and was uncomfortable the entire year. But, I was not in a different one. That was good enough. An unexpected side effect—the dirty desktop used to rub against my belly going up and down and I got grayish stains down the bottom half of my shirts all the time. My mother would ask how I kept getting this specific stain over and over again. I never told her. Some things are best kept to oneself.

Making things much worse was that my personality was the opposite of what my size lead people to expect. Timid, sports hating, non-aggressive, fond of most things girly — this big kid was a big sissy! Teasing intensified. I would be picked on to fight as taking on the biggest kid was many a boy's desire. I flatly refused to fight. Even when they'd hit me, I'd just keep walking away. Taunts being shouted my way. In 2nd grade, I asked my teacher if I could stay in the classroom during recess instead of going out and playing with the other kids. I didn't really like their company. How sad, right? Yes, but I also had an ulterior motive less sympathetic. I'd go through all the kids' lunch boxes and take sweets I wasn't allowed. Remember, my mother disdained all processed stuff. So, pop tarts and Hostess fruit pies and Oreos were contraband I had to devise other ways to get. I learned to sneak very young and got more cunning and bolder with it as my need for more food demanded.

EXAMPLE: I used to lie to my mother that I had to go to the bathroom when we'd be at the supermarket. Then, I'd run down the cake mix aisle and grab the tubes of icing, twist open the cap and SQUEEZE as much of it in my mouth as I could get. Then screw the cap back on, hang it back up and run back, with a tongue some vivid color it shouldn't be. I did this many times.

Don't buy those tubes of icing. A fat kid probably sampled them.

EXAMPLE: One summer, my friend and his family went out of town for a week. I'd seen him take a wrench from their store room, lay on the ground, put his arm up the doggie door to open the front door when he'd forgotten his keys many times. I knew what to do. I went there, got in easily and took advantage of their junk food. On the way home, I reflected. I couldn't believe what I'd just done. But, it worked! When I went back later in the week to do it again, someone was there watering their lawn. Darn it! I pretended I didn't know they were out of town. That's the nature of doing wrong, it gets easier.

EXAMPLE: In 9th grade, I'd had my lunch, but it wasn't enough. I lied to the sweet lady who managed the cafeteria. I said that another kid had stolen my lunch and could I have another one although I didn't have money to pay for one, but I was hungry (insert violin music). She went ballistic! WHO'D dared to take my lunch! She bolted out of the back area in a fury and asked me, in a loud voice, to point out who'd done It. She was going to report them to the principal. I panicked. This was NOT the response I'd expected. I pleaded with her not to do this, it was alright. I calmed her down and that was that. Boy, did that backfire. I think I even passed on another helping. My appetite was gone. A rare feat back then, indeed!

EXAMPLE: As an acolyte, the priest who trained us openly did not like me. I found out later that he was a repressed homosexual and I was obviously gay. Perhaps that's why. Also, world hunger was a focus of our church and he took to it passionately. I seemed to be a physical representative of all that he hated: a fat, gay boy from an upper middle class family that didn't revere his authority. I used to grab all the cookies I could get from the church office tin and run to the bathroom with them. He saw me and pounded on the door for me to come out. He called me a fat pig and insisted that I replace the cookies that I'd taken.

EXAMPLE: While in the church's jurisdiction, there was a doughnut shop across the street and I ate there often. As a new driver, I stopped there to eat 4 or 5 on my way home from school and, gasp, the car didn't start! Not worried about that. I was worried about being at the doughnut shop when I was supposed to be watching my weight. Know what I did? I put that car in neutral, pushed it across the street (traffic, be darned!) to the church parking lot. Then, I called my parents to tell them it wouldn't start and that I'd stopped there to pray. Sorry, God.

My first trip to an organized weight loss program came at age 10. Mother and I joined together. The teacher adored me and I, her. I never forgot one of her funniest one-liners: I love chocolate so much my husband has to hide the Ex-Lax! I got into the diet, to a point. I preferred adults to other children as company already, so being the only kid was no problem. I lost enough weight that other kids at school even commented on it. Diet restricted foods were free game on 'free days'. More or less, I co-operated until I'd come home and they'd be a cake covering the entire kitchen counter. My mother had clearly broken her own diet. That would be that for me, too, then. I only found out later that my father brought this up to her on occasion in private and it lead to arguments. Then he'd drop it. No interest in a lifestyle change at 10. I don't expect kids that age to have foresight or maturity enough to understand health risks or benefits of living well yet. That is the parents' job to lead by example. That didn't happen.

My father's misguided way to straighten me out - weight wise and sissy wise - was to enroll me in sport after sport. None ever took. My 2 years of little league, I didn't fit into the uniforms, so I had to get the closest thing to it from the store. Again, here I am standing out for all the wrong reasons. I know I weighed over 100# at 8 years old as it was loudly announced by the man weighing us for a judo competition. "This boy weighs over 100 pounds" he said as he moved the large weight over one notch on the doctors' scale while all the other kids gawked and gasped. There was no other kid my age anywhere near my size. I was to be matched against a 12-year-old 3 belts higher. I was just going to let him throw me and tap out. They ran out of time and I didn't fight. Whew! No sport really had a chance since I was being forced into them. Well aware of the reasons only made me dig in defiantly even more so. Also, I was well aware my father was embarrassed of his son. I got made fun of by my uncles, cousins, family friends.... all this only drove me to food more. My father and I shared a mutual interest in old movies. I thank God we did as this was our primary bond for many years. Neutral topics were safest.

P.E. was a horrible experience year after year. Running - with my head down heaving = miserable. You had to get weighed for wrestling, that was always humiliating and I would always have to be partnered with a kid older and tougher. Skins versus shirts basketball = horrible. My heart would be pounding with fear at the thought. If I was on a skins team the other kids would laugh at me shirtless. 'Look, he has boobs like a girl!' After a while, I'd say I had to go to the bathroom and just stay there. No one missed me. Oh, how I wanted it to end. Being negatively judged so much since such a big measure of a boy is tied to his athletic prowess. Picked last or next to last for everything or having kids argue over who had to take you. How in the hell was I not supposed to develop a dislike for this? It took me years to even begin to appreciate sports in any way.

Sneaking becomes a necessity when you're addicted to overeating and you're under age. No job, no car, not enough money, having to ask for permission ... DAMN! I couldn't wait to get a job and drive so I could have freedom of choice in these matters. But, for now, I was a sneak master.

EXAMPLE: At the mall, I'd go to 2 different places to have 2 soft serve cones. The chocolate/vanilla combo was mankind's greatest achievement in my mind for many years.

EXAMPLE: I'd get to Junior high school early for the delicious warm sweet rolls. Holy Moly, they were good: gooey, super sweet and cheap. What more could I want? Well, it seems I wanted more of 'em. Lunch time, I'd eat the lunch I'd brought plus milk shakes from the cafeteria. Also, more sweet rolls! Being careful not to go to the line where the kid that had sold me the morning ones was, so they didn't know I was eating 3 and 4 of them a day. They were the only thing in junior high school I truly looked forward to.

EXAMPLE: I lied about my age to get my first job at McDonalds at 15.I looked older and no one doubted me. They kept very tight count on inventory. There were 2 big garbage cans we were to put all mistake foods in one. At the end of the shift, the manager would put on rubber gloves and literally take each messed up thing out of one, count it on an inventory sheet and drop it in the other. If that isn't a point for computers, I don't know what is. After that, we could take the 'mistake trash' out to the dumpster. Oh, I WILL!!!! I'd pull it outside, unpeel burger after burger and create 4 patty gargantuan things that I'd stuff down lukewarm, truly risking choking - I mean eating fast even by MY standards. It was McParadise.

EXAMPLE: Liquor was provided somewhat irresponsibly by today's standards at most parties I attended in high school. Nevertheless, it was the bowl of M and Ms that still engaged me. I'd put handfuls of them in my pockets and lock myself in the bathroom and eat them as fast as I could. I likely had rainbow colored shell in between all my teeth when I emerged. Similar to a drug addict, I suppose.

A diet in the summer, aged 12 or 13, I officially hit 200#. My diet guru also adored me and expressed her disappointment. I'm sure it was out of concern, but I was unreachable. Food was the goal and anyone or anything or anyplace that kept me from it was just getting in my way. I had a one track mind, to say the least. Breakfast was eaten thinking about snacks, eaten while thinking about lunch, eaten while thinking about snacks, eaten while thinking about dinner, eaten while thinking about desserts, eaten while thinking about snacks ... day in and day out - week after week - month after month - year after year.

If you'd think one too many humiliations would do the trick, you'd be logical, but wrong. About 8th grade, I was coming home from school when a man my father hired to help him do some yard work saw me. He asked my father if I was his son. Yes, he replied. "Put a few more pounds on him, he'd make a good sumo wrestler." My dad didn't say

X485

anything. A sumo wrestler - that's how others saw me. Now, I certainly knew I was fat, but somehow hearing that from a stranger rocked me. Somewhere in my head, I fantasized about being a rock star, dance star .... typical teenage stuff. But, this... you know the hardest part: he didn't seem to mean it as an insult. I don't believe he did. He just saw me and put 2 and 2 together. I never forgot that one.

New clothes for high school meant I was aware I had a 48"waist. 'Don't think size, think comfort' the guy at the big man's store said - yeah, yeah, yeah. When the football coaches saw this big guy, something very unexpected happened. I was offered a place on the Varsity football team. I would have been the first freshman in Nevada's history. Oh, HELL no! I didn't even know how to play the game. This would have meant media attention. When I refused the offer, the coaches were so stunned they sent one to my parent's house to explain that I'd be safe. They assumed they objected. It couldn't have come from me. This unprecedented opportunity turned down by a 14-year-old boy!? I became one of the managers of the team in my sophomore year to get a letterman's jacket. Easier!

Towards the end of my freshman year, I went to Overeaters Anonymous. Just turned 15, it was the first time I'd heard people approach what I was doing as an addiction. Similar to alcohol, smoking, gambling and drugs - you can be addicted to overeating. I connected with it deeply and for the first time in my life, got very serious about losing weight. The original program was called gray sheet - the foods you were to eat from were printed on a gray sheet. It was very restrictive and based on the fact that you simply need to eat to live. Not live to eat. Food was to be nothing more. I bonded with my sponsor and called her daily to report my eating. I lost 110 or 115 pounds in 5 months and returned to school my sophomore year a different person. I was the talk of the school. Everyone admired what I'd done. They were shocked. It was like no other feeling I'd ever experienced. I bought clothes from normal stores in normal sizes for the first time. That was great fun. I went to OA meetings and they stood and applauded for me.

Alas, this euphoria was not to last. Like the football situation, I didn't realize the enormous amount of attention this would bring could have unwanted consequences. Being thin now meant I was expected to play sports! The excuse of being too fat was gone. I still didn't want to. Also, being thin meant I would receive attention from girls. I knew I was gay, as did most everyone. But now it was official. If I didn't have a girlfriend, this disco dancing, non football playing, old movie watching guy was 100% fag. This brought teasing back just like in grammar school. Wow, I was disillusioned!

With that, my determination waned. I gave in to temptation for the first time in the longest stretch I'd ever had with a fast food hamburger and threw up from it quickly. My system had been cleansed of that nasty stuff and it didn't thank me for re-introducing it. But, that's the nature of yo-yo dieting. Your body gets accustomed to both with enough tenacity! My remaining high school years, I kept my weight relatively in some control fluctuating about 30 pounds or so. That only meant I had to keep 2 sizes of everything. By Christmas, I'd be tightly in the bigger pants and back on a diet and they'd sort of fit again. I'd simply eat next to nothing for a few days and off the pounds went. Of course, this syndrome feeds off itself by its extreme nature.

Social events were curtailed by my ever present desire for more food. But, my high school years kept me watching my weight because I did want to participate in the experience. I managed to be the always nice guy who was in no clique but most people's friends. This was my perfect niche. No dating, as I was a sort of asexual good guy who never pushed himself on anyone. I got on well enough with the kids that I was elected school senator 3 years! Imagine that! Also, I loved to dance all my life and belonged to a little pop group we had. We were very good. I wasn't the strongest link, perhaps, but I showed up on time, pitched in when there was work to be done and sang tenor well enough. We won a state competition my senior year. High school had to end, though.

College brought more than the expected 'freshman 15'. The buffet nature of the dining commons was about as helpful as allowing an alcoholic to keep inventory control over the booze. I had little to no direction for a career because my fixation on food was all that truly interested me. I was bullied on campus for being gay and my one friend and I were ostracized everywhere we went. It was a horrible experience that permanently soured me on college. I know it contributed to me never getting a degree. After my first year, I moved back East to live with my parents. I attended a local state college half-heartedly. I was very unhappy about being gay, overweight, direction- less and my future, in general. This led me to therapy. It would prove to be an unfruitful endeavor I kept for a few years off and on. I never was fully candid about what I was going through, mostly because I didn't like what I was really thinking. #1 – I'm gay, no doubt about it, but scared and unhappy about it. #2 - Frankly, all I care about is eating. Just couldn't bring myself to say that out loud.

My biggest fun was being a bus boy at a coffee shop in a hotel in Atlantic City. I was eating as much food as I could. Employee cafeteria meals before, during and after work - why not! A roll shoved in while I prepared your order— fine! I ran my but off, and I ate off customer's plates what they didn't finish if I wanted it. Classic story: There was a fire alarm during my shift and we all had to evacuate the premises. The boardwalk we all went to was pitch black. I'd taken a steak off a plate and ate it out there with my bare hands. Just tearing it up like an animal. Thank GOD I had my towel in my apron pocket. I probably had blood on my face. When we were allowed back in, the diner said, 'Someone took my steak!' Wow, who'd do something like that? Now, pardon me while I floss.

Better still, the manager put me in charge of the pastry cart - what! I ordered all the sweets, taking freely of them for my own consumption. I could walk down a flight of stairs holding a tray full of sweets in one arm while I devoured an éclair with the other. Never dropped a speck!! I had to go back to the uniform department for bigger pants and a shirt in less than a year. When I needed bigger ones still, I was too ashamed to go back again. My solution - my apron covered me from the second shirt button down to my thighs - yippee! I could leave the shirt unbuttoned and brought safety pins to keep it attached to my pants. They stayed up and I got a diamond of room for my expanded belly and on the feeding could go. Genius!

Personally, I also decided I couldn't deal with being gay. I'd had a couple of brief experiences and didn't seem cut out for it. I decided to be celibate. Now, with no vices to indulge in (I didn't smoke, gamble, do drugs, drink or have sex now added to it) and a decision to remain that way, my food fixation only deepened. I simply didn't care anymore. At 23, I was free. Meaning, with all I wasn't going to do, I was damn well gonna eat whatever I wanted. For the next decade, I did. My weight exploded. I ate with total abandon and no apologies or explanations about the diet I would begin soon. This was a new low. No lip service to any other plan. It was all about food. 250-275— 300 ugh! My 20s were basically wasted. The 1980s: not my decade.

Jobs were just something to endure because we all have to pay rent or mortgage, put gas in a car, see an occasional movie - nothing else. I couldn't have been more out of place in the yuppie decade of 'you can have it all' thinking. I didn't want it all. Want it all, ha! I only wanted one thing - more food! Careers were a waste of time. They take wardrobes, ambition, require you to focus on other things like having a college degree or learning a trade, you have to be looking for the next step up for more work, travel, assignments, pressure.... I wasn't interested. A job was all I could be bothered with. Those other people were fools. It was very disconcerting to see my high school class mates coming back from college with degrees and getting married and such at a time when I wasn't even out of the starting gate. I lost touch with them very quickly. You have to have a vague idea of where you're charging towards to successfully launch. I was happy being an obese slacker on the sidelines. Ferdinand the bull wants to smell the flowers and eat, thank you very much.

For my sister's wedding, when I went to the tuxedo rental place they were laughing. What at? There was one 60" pair of pants the company had that were shipped to various stores this chain had throughout the East coast. They were holding them up and gawking - oh, my God, LOOK at these? Who could be this fat? I would one day be that size.

Relationships were also not for me. I thought they were for fools, too. All that blah, blah, blah talk I'd hear at work about so and so's boyfriends, girlfriends, wife, husbands, dates that didn't go well... ... who needed it? Waste of time and effort, if you ask me. Why didn't they see it? Food was my lover. Food demanded all my time, dedication, money and anyone else was an obstacle to endure. I was known by my first name at 7-11s for my super big gulp of coke I got every morning at 6am, at Burger King for my double whopper and large fries, at Baskin

Robbins for hand packed pints and at JoJo's for peach melbas. I had to keep change on me at all times because vending machines didn't begin to accept dollar bills until the 1990s. My candy bar habit was endless. I never outgrew anything I liked as a kid. I wondered why so many did. At the before mentioned teenage parties where the other kids were focused on the beer or the opposite sex, I was still ogling the goodies. I loved my millionth doughnut, candy bar, cookie, burrito, pie, cake and all other forms of gluttony I've occupied my life with as much as the first one. I can't explain it.

I reacquainted myself with a dear friend via a chance meeting in a used record store in 1990 and it greatly redirected my life. We'd known each other from grade school through high school, were both gay and kindred spirits with a love for old movies, dancing and equal disdain for all things math, sports and domestically conventional. He was very easy going, had made it big as a dancer, very fit and socially outgoing. He insisted I go out with him and I began exploring life as a gay man sincerely for the first time. Funny thing, some men like big men. And that's what they got when they saw me. 300# became 325. 48" waists become 50"! Oh, wow. I went out, danced, and even got hit on. I couldn't believe it. I never followed through. But it was flattering to be asked. My libido has never been very high even in what is supposed to be a man's peak years of late adolescence to early 20s. My self-esteem must have been more intact than I'd known. A fat fetishist would not get their way with me.

My job in a hotel was mundane but very secure. My seniority ensured I could probably stay there forever if I so desired. All back-of-the-house, repetitious paper work, no advancements, you could eat at your desk, nearly everyone there was overweight. It was a perfect job for an ambition-less obese man who needed to make a living. Huge soda pops on the way to work, croissandwiches from Burger King for breakfast, candy bars from the vending machine, more soda pops .... all this was a daily morning routine. I'd walk past the health spa and see the vacationers exercising and say to myself, "Idiots! You're on holiday!" Later, I would be one of them. But that was much later. Lunch - any junk in the cafeteria and LOTS of it. Big helpings of lasagna with mounds of parmesan cheese, two knockwursts piled with everything that would stay on, sandwiches piled with so much peanut butter it tasted like I was swallowing tablespoons of paste (in fact, isn't that exactly what I WAS doing?). Also, I was an expert at stacking desserts onto one platter for the sake of space. On the way home, often a drive through at Jack in the box for a burger and fries to be consumed while I was in the car. I am well aware I had an angel overlooking me when I drove because I regularly ate to distraction while driving. I'm sure I was leaning over for that final extra crispy burnt fry many times without paying a bit of attention to the road. How I didn't kill someone is amazing. Next, a gargantuan dinner in or out would follow a few hours later and always a very high calorie sweet at the end. Later that night, a pint of Hagen Daaz or four pop tarts.... Every day was pretty much like that. It was all about eating. On my days off, I'd fix a box of pasta, a family size jar of sauce, and piles of parmesan cheese, and eat it off my belly with a serving spoon. I'd gorge until I'd puke. Then, I'd be glad for the room in my belly that vomiting provided so I could continue eating.

Don't misunderstand. I'm not proud of any of this. It came with many miserable consequences. My chair at the table had to be armless. There was never a matching proper set in our dining room. I had to sit only at tables in restaurants because booths were simply impossible. I broke the alignment of my aforementioned friend's dad's car due to my weight. It made grinding noises the day after we'd been out in it. When he took it to the repair shop, the mechanic asked him how the front passenger side had broken. Did they try to move a large piece of furniture or a refrigerator? No, only massive me. He didn't tell his dad the real reason.

I found out seatbelt extenders were available on airplanes. I wish I'd known sooner. When my weight left me unable to buckle the seatbelt I tucked it under my track suit. I was so scared they had some sort of monitoring devices and would confront me while everyone looked on. I was literally sweating with fear over this: a new low. No meal for me because the tray didn't come down due to my huge belly. What irony.

Only elastic on all pants is pretty much mandatory after a certain size since my fluctuations were so wild it wasn't possible to function any other way. Buttons, belts, zippers, non-elastic pants…the enemy! Perhaps most alarming of all of these was waking up in the middle of the night with a numb right arm. That was fun. A warning of an impending stroke at 32. I could go on and on here. But I've made my point.

Eventually 400#... WOW. I weigh more than 400#. As is the insidious nature of gluttony and obesity, there is no top number. The same simple cycle went on. 400 became 420. A 54" waist became 56. My mother would occasionally express concern about how big I was going to let myself get. Hard to believe, but my answer to her was the truth most of the time; I really didn't think about it too much. If I did, I'd want to kill myself. Oh, and don't think I was so blind I was unaware of the massive health risks I was taking. I just didn't care. What kind of life did I need to stick around 50 more years for? Only food mattered and there was a price to pay for how I ate and I paid it. 420 became 440. 56" waist became 58".

When I saw photos of myself, I would sometimes get the reality check of just how huge I was. I would be standing next to regular sized people and literally see myself at two, three and four times their size. This didn't please me. It would hurt. Not enough to do anything constructive about it for an awfully long time, though. I had managed to succeed at a job (two times employee of the month), to my amazement had a small group of friends and ate whatever the **** I wanted. For more than 10 years I had lived the dream (my version), until I saw it as the nightmare it had long become.

It took some health scares to make me even consider reassessing myself. I could not walk well. I didn't recognize myself in the mirror. My forearm looked like a normal person's leg. My sleep was disturbed greatly. I broke furniture and cars. Clothes wore out due to sweat and friction regularly. My mother told me of a surgery being tested called a gastro intestinal bypass. It was for people like me in my situation: morbidly obese patients who are unable to control their eating. I was interested enough to attend a seminar given by the sole doctor in Nevada at the time who was launching this procedure. Indeed, the stomach is stapled and a tube is attached to the smaller portion and re-attached someplace in the middle of the intestines to bypass much of the digestion / calorie absorption. For good measure, a silastic ring would be placed on the bottom of my esophagus to further limit my eating to miniscule bites. I'm surprised how open to this radical undertaking I was. It just seemed to be well timed. My mother was equally surprised how willing I was to do this. In 1995, at 33, I was weighed at a loading dock in the back of the hospital at my top weight of 485. I was in 62 / 64" pants and size 4XL or 5XL shirts. Pushing 500# and almost to the top size even big men's stores carried. If I gained much more I'd have had to have my clothes custom tailored: another new low to experience.

In this sorry state, I became one of the first people in the state of Nevada to get this surgery. I came through it rather well. No doubt, due to my youth, I'd managed to come out of my years of self- abuse with little damage. I'm very lucky, it could have gone very, very badly. The initial withdrawal was like a cold bucket of water. It was over. I could not overeat again. We pioneers met at a weekly support group. I cried that I regretted doing this. The reality hit me: eating slowly, small bites, putting forks down would all have to be regular parts of my life. The surgery is irreversible. There is no changing your mind, unhappy or not. No surprise, my weight dropped dramatically. For about 8 months or so, my body was adjusting internally and my appetite and digestion were just not there. Was this truly the magic the world was waiting for?

I'm sure you know there's no such thing as magic. At group we all lamented our private trials. The throwing up, the foods you can't tolerate forever, the isolation you didn't count on, the gas unfiltered digestion gives.... worst, there is no mental preparing for life. Worse still, the tool could be 'gotten around'! I don't know if the doctors genuinely didn't know this at this early stage or felt it was best to not fully inform us. The stomach is a very stretchy organ that has the ability to adapt and you could overeat again. Not as fast and nowhere near the same portions at one time that you were having previously. But, if it's your intention, you could undo all the benefits. People could regain the weight!

While still in the losing and unable to overeat stage, I had to have 2 follow up reconstructive plastic surgery procedures for the layers of skin. This was less vanity and more of a necessity. I was fileted like a fish. Fortunately, I'm very hairy and the scars don't show much. I also had a nose job thrown in while I was under the knife. I'd never had a flat chest or stomach my entire life. It was like looking at another person's body when I looked in the mirror.

In 2 years' time, I took off over 200#. When I first went under 300#, it was the first time in at least 8 years. Everyone I saw who'd known me commented on my massive weight loss. At work, at church, at the DMV, neighbors ... everyone I'd ever been in contact with. It was like sophomore year on steroids. It was like a dream, again. Dreams don't last. My mental behavior wasn't fixed. There wasn't a miracle transformation. As I'd said, knowledge of post-surgical life wasn't available at the time.

EXAMPLE: There is the spitting up you cannot control. I have to eat meals with a cup in case I unintentionally regurgitate. This is like King Midas' dilemma. Everything can make you throw up. Unpleasant and very socially limiting, I have to be extremely cautious in public.

EXAMPLE: Your body readjusts and you can eat more, then more. You may get sick, but if you KEEP DOING IT, that gets better, too. Now, if that isn't a picture of an addict, I don't know what is. We were told if we drank soda pop that would send us to the emergency room. Still, nearly all of us tried It. Some couldn't take it, others could. I am fine with it. I drink pop to this day. Unintentionally perhaps, but I began to undo all of the benefits I'd experienced. I COULD eat again, so I DID eat again. In 1995, I weighed 485. In 1997 I weighed 220 or so. By late 1998, I was back at 270 again.

I cannot fully express my shock, shame and utter despair. My surgeon was not equipped for the backsliding many of the patients were having and dissembled the support group. At my final meeting with him, he told me he was giving up on me. I was a hopeless case whom he predicted would regain all the weight and die. I didn't feel like that was the ending I was after. Now what? In 1998, what I'd had done was literally the end of the road. There wasn't anything else (at least not known to the general public). If this didn't work, I was beyond helping. This was one of my life's lowest points.

Well, what to do now? I was dropped by my physician and didn't want to regain all the weight. I went to a diet doctor for some pills. He was a nice enough guy. Not pushy, usually those types are. He was selling appetite suppressants that were going to have side effects and cost $200+ a month. I took his card and pamphlet and left. When my mother saw them, I told her where I'd been and she suggested going back on another program. 'Oh, no, I've tried over and over. It doesn't work!' I said. She replied, 'You joined all those times. You never really DID it.' I stood frozen. This was the closest I'd ever come to magic in my life. The moment was a magic bullet. I don't know exactly why that statement hit me so, but it did. Some of you know there can be moments between you and your mother where she says something you don't like but you both KNOW is true. I couldn't say a word. We were both there. There was no denying it. Not even a convenient 3rd person in the room I could deflect this annoying truth to and divert it somewhat. "What do you think of that?" 3rd person: "Leave me OUT of this!" She was right. I knew it. I would try again…thank you, mother.

My mother and I were always very close. It was difficult for me to type words of blame on her in the early part of this story. It was true. She did put me on the path to overeating. She was in the grasp of it herself. A drowning person can't save another drowning person. She told me many times of her tremendous guilt for putting me on the path that consumed me and nearly killed me. As an adult, I firmly believe one's sins, foibles, trials … all become your own. You simply cannot remain stagnant all your life because of how you were raised. I had to rise to that occasion. She'd tried over and over again to help me. I have her to thank for finding the surgery as I certainly wasn't looking. I have her to thank for guiding me back to watching my weight with the right mind set. Both would save my life. So, in the redemption line, she did a 2-for-1 for herself. I forgive any and all of my mother's errors or lapses in judgment regarding my upbringing 100%. Long ago, I did this. I made my own miserable years for myself. She did her best and was the best mother I've ever seen.

I, too, forgive my father. He had had a very difficult upbringing and didn't know how to help me, either. Pushing me into sports was tremendously damaging and he didn't mean anything but well. I now believe this. I didn't for many years. You cannot expect any more out of someone than the best they can do. He got nicer as he aged. Our relationship deepened as adults. I was a comfort to him and he began to realize the benefits of having a gay son. I would always be there for the two of them in a way you can't be if you marry, move away and start your own family. We became pals. He was a better father than most I've seen.

Trying to lose weight for the umpty-umpth time in early 1999, I always say spiritually it was my first time. It was different than all the others. I had the proper attitude. So, I had everything. Nevertheless, I still ate 2 cherry Hostess fruit pies on my way to join the program. All changes in their time. But, I truly didn't just want to lose weight ... again. I wanted to treat it like a permanent lifestyle change. This was new, indeed. I wanted to do it! Wow, what a new color this was. Amazing, I did the program as it was explained by my teacher eagerly. Even the day after my weigh in wasn't a free day. This had long been a typical thing for me. Of COURSE, the next day was a free day. That often extended much longer. I took off 100# for a life total of 300#! This has stayed off, for the most part - life still provides struggles - for over 16 years from 485 to 185.

To be sure, I'm much prouder of the maintaining of the loss than I am the losing. Anyone can lose weight temporarily. For longer, only a life-style change works. My father passed away unexpectedly in 1996. He saw me initially losing my weight on the first go around, but never saw me thin. I would have loved that. A dream came true when I reached goal when I was able to wear an all-white outfit. White is my favorite color. It is the least slimming color. One of my desires was to be slim and able to look good in white top to bottom. I'll never forget standing in that dressing room with white button fly Levi's and a size medium white ribbed cotton shirt I tucked in. I checked myself out mercilessly from all angles in that dressing room. Lean to the left, the right, pre-tend to pick something up and look at my white butt, squat ... you get it: a very thorough exam. When I realized I looked alright, I got very emotional. "Yes! Yes! Yes! Yes! YES!" I stood there and thought I've waited 30+ years for this moment. You don't get too many opportu-nities to have one precise moment where you can say that. It was a moment I'll never forget.

As I got close to goal, my teacher informed me that I was going to become a teacher. Honestly, I hadn't considered it. But, I was an obe-dient student and simply pursued this at her insistence. This would be something new. I hadn't had a public contact job in over a dozen years and even then it wasn't as public as this. The training was putting me into an entirely different field than I'd ever experienced. I've read that speaking in public is the greatest fear for most people - more than sharks, diseases or death. Well, here I was doing just that - and loving it. too! I began part time to see if I had a knack for it. Turns out, I did!

You can train, but there is a part that can't be taught. It's either there or it isn't. This is very true with public speaking. I was helping others suffering and came alive off their energy and successes.

Oh, THIS is what it feels like to get up and enjoy your work! I hadn't had that feeling. I was accustomed to enduring my job, living for my days off, wishing my life away. This glimpse of another way made my full time job unbearable. My attitude turned poor towards it. I was always a very good employee. My boss was an overweight eating partner of mine whom I know didn't like the new me as much as the obese me. The obese me worked any shift, days off changed, trained clerks with no title or compensation, came early, left late, cut lunch hours short .... was as hard working and reliable an employee as you could want. My reward: a clerk for 13 years and I expected to be fired all the time. What food is worth that?

Now, I'd tasted a new life and I left my job of 15 years without a backwards glance for an uncertain future spreading the gospel of health, weight loss and only receive commission that would not be reliable in an untried position. I was a test rabbit as the program's first full time leader in the state of Nevada and one of the few males ever, too. It turned out spectacularly. The more I felt bright and happy, the brighter my clothes got. I'm known for my bold, bright, over the top wardrobe. I don't need to pay a therapist to see how the pendulum swung the other way after years of having to wear drab clothes from the big man's store - black, brown, slate gray, dark navy, tan - ugly, ugly, ugly. Now, head to toe purple, just another day at the office. Loud golf pants in the wildest styles - John Daly shouldn't get all the fun! Hounds tooth slacks in bright yellow and black - ring it up!!

Seriously, seeing others who are wounded and suffering recover and discover their true self and the quality of life they can have and be free from the chains their extra weight forces them to bear makes mine the most rewarding job I can imagine. In the many years I've been doing it, it's no less joyous. It was the bravest risk I've ever taken and it's been my honor and privilege ever since meeting all the people who look to me to help them on their own journey to their own happy ending. You'll soon read some of their stories.

One final thing - you're never cured. Never. I still struggle every day to do what I can to resist returning to my old ways. I always tell beginners I didn't get thin because I woke up one day and decided ice cream doesn't taste good anymore and I lived happily ever after. Though that'd make a KILLER ending, it wouldn't be true. Don't people actually eat pizza folded in half so they can shovel in more, faster? Who knew! I am only caging my beast and he wants to get out all the time. I accept this burden and I bear it to the best of my ability all the time. Oh, and keeping weight off only gets harder as you age. I am always only giving it my best one day at a time. Food remains the top focus of my life and potential nemesis. It probably will be until I take my final breath. Realistic expectations can bring peace of mind. So I fight, and fight, and fight. Is it worth it? Abso- frickin-lutely!

PROLOGUE PROFILES:

Book knowledge is necessary, vital and in our ever revolving society, continually changing. The mere recollection of some of my sad, desperate, embarrassing things I've done in the name of food could fill volumes. But, still, be only one person's story.

Why aren't we all thin and healthy? Certain truths are basic regarding weight loss and maintaining it. But we must admit: Fattening foods taste great! Great is too weak a word for it. People who are non-food obsessed confuse me. What's wrong with them? Can I please have your secret?

Interacting with literally thousands of people has given me a wide perspective. Knowledge is absorbed, applied, modified, toyed with and utterly ignored on a person by person basis. By our nature, we crave pleasure. Eating brings tremendous pleasure. It can distort our thinking. It can make us lie, conceal, spend money foolishly, litter, force ourselves to purge, take on health risks that range from silly to fatal. Then, pass these on to our kids. Human beings require food. Like sleep and breathing, it's a body function. In America, the obesity epidemic has only gotten worse in the years I've been working. The gap is getting wider with the next generation. Try as I do, if the individual isn't a fully co-operative partner in this, nothing will work for too long. I wanted this book to reflect that.

What you're going to read is a collection of stories of 40 students I've met in my career as a weight loss counselor. They are a varied bunch picked for their unique journeys. After a lifetime battle with obesity, I'd gotten myself thin and felt a calling to bring the message of weight loss to all who suffered and were willing to change. I quit my job of more than 15 years and haven't looked back. It's very rewarding work. As much as I try to give to my students, they give me more than I could ever return.

These students, regular people from all walks of life, valiantly attempt to re-arrange food's place in their lives. You will get brief glimpses into their journey. Bullet points to take lessons from. They play out in many directions. A few do not have happy endings. For privacy protection, names and some minor details have been changed. Nothing omitted was of any importance for what you're meant to learn. There are victories, glorious conquering heroes and heroines who've done what they'd thought could never happen. I, myself, consider the very top accomplishment the maintaining of the weight loss. No doubt.

There are those who lost the weight and took their eyes away from the rigorous work that got them there. The floodgates of regression catch them back and a re-climbing of the mountain must be begun. Perhaps they're tempered and wiser and willing to not repeat past errors.

Our country may not be fully in sync with my approach. I am not a computer person: online diets and apps seem to be the future. They've taken a big bite out of my class attendance. I am a people person - hands on, eye to eye, face to face is my style. It seems to be the old fashioned way now. Pity, I still believe in it. Computer tools are useful, yes. But when I'm told they're replacing traditional classes, I must object. This trend is becoming the new normal. Will the next generation only know internet learning? I got a flash of this at the dentist when the 20 something girl asked me 'What do you go to a class for?' She didn't mean to be rude. She was genuinely unaware of why one would physically **go** to a center and interact with people when there are 100s of apps for weight loss.

Some profiles are of those who did not succeed. Why did I include them? I stewed about this. But I felt it was important to shine a light on my years doing this as realistically as possible. This book is called 'Confessions of a weight loss counselor'. It is not exclusively a 'self-help' / 'how-to' book in the instructional sense. You must hear and can learn from the non-achievers, too.

All have an Epilogue of sorts called Tips and Traps. The primary points to retain while translating their stories into your own game plan are highlighted and explained a bit further. Read them as you would speak to a friend. These good people deserve that from you.

Life is stranger than fiction. You can't make this stuff up. I hope by reading this, you make a decision to take your life and health in hand. Just a small group of short stories - but they represent more than a decade of work. Make a decision and you're more than 1/2 way there. I made a decision years ago - no matter how much the world may give up on being thin, I will not. We have bigger plates, movie theater chair arms lift, sizes in department stores have been increased to accommodate the larger size of the patrons, and we get less and less active. But I will fight against it - even if I am a solitary warrior on one side of the mountain, I'll go out swinging. Join me.

1—Mike

2 —Joyce

3— How long is this gonna take?

4—Zack and Anne

5—Tina

6—Yvonne and Joe

7—Misty

8— Opal and Laura

9—Adam

10 — Claire

11— Charlotte

12— Olivia

13— Guy and Nora

14— Kelly

15—Larry

16— Vicki

17— Ashley

18—Zelda

19— Ken

20— Money matters

21—Wanda

MIKE:

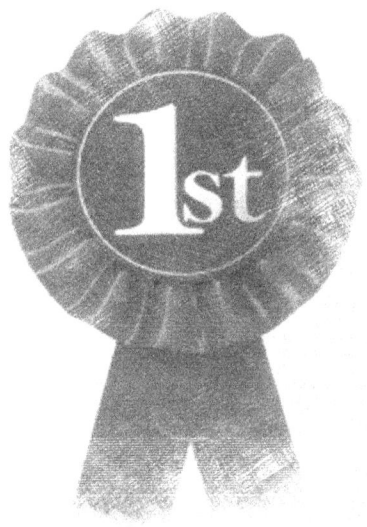

Mike was a character. I've been called a character all my life, too. Perhaps that's why we took to each other so well: kindred spirits. Time would prove this most true. Tall, bald, Hawaii shirt wearing Mike strolled into a meeting of mine and informed me that he was a lapsed member who'd been overweight all his life, like me, and had been on every variation the program had, like me. His fluctuations were massive: another shared trait. We gained and lost 100+# the way some people do 20 or 30. You have to have lived with this type of obesity and food obsession to this degree to fully understand it. We took to our similar circumstances, bonded and Mike engaged.

Further to my surprise (Mike is a never ending genie bottle of surprises); he told me he used to work for the program back in the day. He didn't take to the bosses and didn't stay with it too long. But, wow, and how did he stand the previous program he'd been most successful with? One difference, I liked the new program much more that the older ones. Mike was looking backwards a bit. That was part of his dilemma. I could help him with that.

It's an albatross that distracts many former members if they're married to a past diet. If they'd been successful at it, I do understand the reluctance to release it. But, it is necessary or you're always looking backwards, never fully applying yourself to the current program and not getting the weight off. Then, it can further deepen the belief that the old way is not to be messed with and they don't get the support they came to the classes for. No, that won't do. I tell people to shake the Etch-a- Sketch of the past before they go forward as a physical and spiritual cleansing of it. They all have a 100% clear shot at every new try. Thank goodness this is true. As a multi repeater, I wouldn't have made it if it were not true. Yesterday needs to stay in the rear view.

Mike's grandkids were his primary motivation. He clearly loved them and any mention of them melted away his slick persona often to the point of tears. Mike was from a small town, busted out, moved to the big city and led an adventurous life with myriad accomplishments. His conversations are engaging and he has a natural ability to attract people to him. It's a gift we share. You can't earn a living talking to people without it, really. Months would pass and another subject would come up and he'd have the coolest story about it. What hasn't Mike done? Climb Mt Everest? Maybe he has.

A life-long lover of healthy food and exercise were two HUGE legs up for Mike. Oh, how he'd play with the pun level of that statement. I can hear it now! They served him well. In fact, his food habits were so sound I wondered how he'd gotten overweight in the first place. He loved fruit, veggies, seafood, water, brown rice and took vitamins like a scholar. He didn't eat red meat, full fat dairy, and junk food or was very sweet toothed. So, how did his weight ever become a problem?

In a word: bread. Mike was a bread-a-holic. I shouldn't have been surprised at that when he said he wasn't into sugar. I am addicted to it. I could inject Hershey's syrup into my veins, it's that bad. When I meet people who confess they genuinely are not into sweets, it's usually carbs that did them in. I am not into carbs. We are on opposite sides of the fence on that: potato chips, bread, crackers.... not my addiction. I don't hate them, but they don't bother me. It would be a fun meeting, albeit an unproductive one, to tell our favorite temptations and let others raise their hands if that food isn't the slightest problem for them. We'd all gasp and say, 'How's that possible? What wrong with you?' and laugh. Mike often dined on entire two-foot-long baguettes of bread. How did he get the protruding stomach in the before picture he proudly displayed now that is was gone? The answer: bread, chips, et al. Oh, and a full stick of butter slathered over it. Well, that'd do it. No box of doughnuts or pints of ice cream for this guy. But, what's the difference. Obesity doesn't discriminate. Mike often joked that he looked nine months pregnant at his highest.

As is often the case with funny folks, there was a sad cover up underneath. He'd been an overweight child and took many scars to his adult life with it. This was another way we'd bonded. I share my many scars life as an overweight kid and teen often in meetings. It helps people know that behind my smiling goofy attired persona are many years of suffering and hard knocks. Mike was a slick talking, supremely confident guy with a sewed together heart. His children brought out the softer side. His wife and daughters were overweight. They'd passed on the unhealthy habits to the next generation and they were certainly enduring the life it entails now. Mike was trying to help them in any way he could. But this is a journey no one can take for you. I, too, had come from an overweight home and had my parents try to help me without me fully engaged. It didn't work for me. It doesn't work for anyone until they're fully on board. Mikes' kids were no exceptions… back to Mike.

He was fearless in his professional life, enjoyed a healthy social life, travelled often, was liberal in his thinking, and enjoyed opera. No wonder he didn't fit in in small town, USA. He was meant to travel the world. Well, only the tropical parts. Mike hates the cold.

Not only did Mike lose 120+# for the third time, but he did it with grit, determination, and while he shows the world his 'mask of aplomb', I know he worked VERY hard for it. Mike's wife passed away while on his losing journey. If there's a reason you could use to regain your weight and no one object, that'd be it. Not Mike. He shared his obvious heartbreak with the room, but kept going. His healthy turn around had not been shared with his wife, so his golden years will not be shared with her, either. So sorry, Mike, so very sorry.

His dedication to exercise kept him much healthier than his eating habits would have had him at his age. Exercise and its benefits score another one! Mike is determined to dance at his grandkids' weddings. It's his focus. Maintaining weight loss is very difficult and Mike struggles with it. Despite his arguing to the contrary, he is not Superman. He is a real hero, instead. One I am truly blessed to know.

Proof of the kind of man and friend he is has been shown to me and many over and over again. He will be dancing at all his grandkid's life milestones with that twinkle of mischief in his eye as surely as I type this.

TIPS: Communicate with your counselors, teachers and coaches. Those willing to be taught will be taught. Mike came to learn. His open mind was fertile ground teachers can work with. How is yours? Reexamine it. If you're reachable, then you're teachable.

TRAPS: Mike's rocket ride to goal idled when a new relationship began. A social lady who entertained very graciously and often, there were many food temptations. Mike's focus was diverted. Extensive travel further scrambled it. I'm sure Mike would have recaptured goal by now if he'd been uninterrupted. Will new people in your life distract you?

JOYCE:

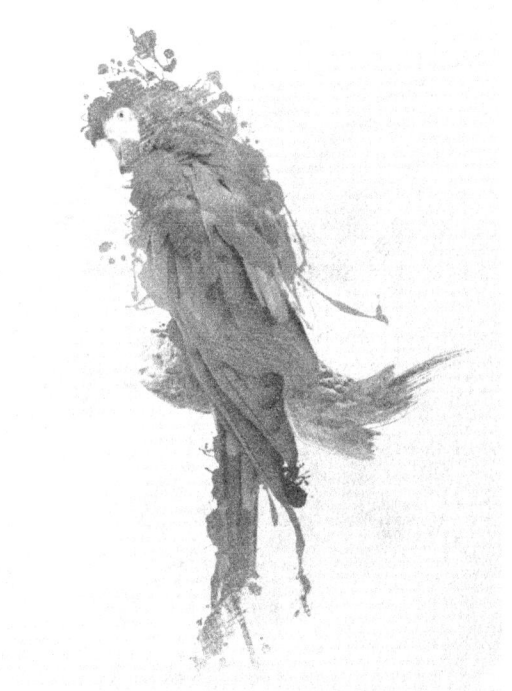

Joyce, once you've met her, you don't forget her. Some would call her loud, brash, déclassé, tacky and unrefined. They'd all be right. Joyce didn't dress to impress, either. Off the shoulder elastic was a staple of her wardrobe. Also, she liked bike shorts - the tighter, the better. Joyce liked the sun a lot, too. No worries about skin damage for this deeply bronzed lady. Mouthwash was also not used. Hairspray, on the other hand, was used generously. High, country style! Just about everything I have said is why we became fast friends. Really, some of us are just a bit 'off', me, included. We want to be treated with respect and kindness and accepted as we are, just like everybody. I could tell she was in need of a lot of that. I'd see to it she got plenty.

More than 100# overweight and only 5'3", Joyce was getting to the point where the burden of all this excess strain was wearing her down. Upbeat in personality and gregarious, being unable to get where she wanted to go didn't suit Joyce. In her younger days, she'd dragged herself around better than most. Unfortunately, sometimes when there aren't any 'in your face' negative side effects, some people ignore the problem. Until it becomes one, that is. Well, now it was. Joyce was also a smoker and her time pushing the envelope was running out. That is why she joined the program.

Joyce had a husband, kids, a job, family and liked to socialize and exercise. I could work with this one. Exercise had paid off for her. As I said, she was the fastest walking, most active 100+# person I've met and I've met hundreds. In her 40s, she still wanted to be active and avoid any illnesses getting in her way. She only informed me to leave her cigarettes out of it. She wasn't quitting that AND this. I complied with her wishes. A life-long non-smoker who was surrounded by many smokers, they'd turned me off completely. Not even a single puff has been taken into my lungs. I say this to justify my leaving her smoking be. I don't know what nicotine addiction feels like. Therefore, I'm unqualified to coach anyone on it in any personal way. I've read stories of rock stars that have beaten heroin, cocaine and alcoholism that say they can't stop. Fine, I was going to help Joyce get thin.

The program was taken in with little resistance. Joyce was truly ready. As a fellow member of the 100+# overweight club, I could virtually write her stats on how she ate. What unhealthy thing didn't she eat? It was as though she'd compiled a list of every fattening junk you could eat or drink and stuck with that. She jogged miles on a stationary bike, took aerobics classes, lifted weights, power walked, country-line danced, swam and was interested in any new popular contraption her gym had. She heard many comments from her fellow gym mates about how mysterious it was that she was so big when she worked out so hard, harder than most of them did. Well, you can unravel anything if that's your aim. It'd been Joyce's aim. We needed to redirect her.

Making all that valiant effort NOT pay off is a task unto itself. As I said, from the mornings full of bacon, butter loaded toast and Pop tarts to lunches of any kind of fast food or deep fried option closest to where she worked to snacking on Dolly Madison cakes throughout the day to dinners of epic portions of gravy drenched meat loafs, potatoes made unrecognizable under the dollops of sour cream, bacon and cheese and ending evenings with pints of the fullest fat ice creams covered in gooey sauces. Yea, that could do it.

Oh, AND smoking. No amount of Olympian efforts would've kept the fat off. It's the only reason she wasn't 200+# overweight.

Happily, Joyce took to healthy food better than I'd expected. There's often a period of withdrawal that takes a lot of will power to overcome. I have failed at this initial shock to the body adjustment many times. It can be really tough. Joyce took it in stride. She was very determined. Turkey bacon, ok, low fat milk, sure, butter buds, yes, lean cuts of meat, no problem, veggies, after I figure out how to cook 'em, I'll eat 'em, salad not drowned in dressing, wow, it's supposed to be green! Every salad I'd ever eaten was white or orange, sugar free puddings, not bad, lite beer, cheers! Joyce impressed me.

In the gym, she discovered that healthy fuel in her body made for phenomenal energy. She was already a leader in the place, but now she could run it! Motivation has to be personal for it to have any hope of being permanent. I cannot give it to anyone. We all have to discover it for ourselves. Joyce had high standards for fitness. She realized she'd been tackling these obstacles with a 100+# back pack on without really knowing it. Now that it was off, look out! Eat Joyce's dust, everyone!

She'd show up for class earlier than the doors were even unlocked, sit right on the ground and light up a smoke. Joyce was nobody's idea of a proper lady. When I'd open the door, I'd say, 'Aren't you hot?' and she'd act like it was a silly question. She was fine, nothing to worry about. She liked waiting on the ground. O-K, Joyce. Sometimes she'd have bags of canned food from her bargain hunts. Proudly she'd tell the class about the different church's outreach pantries and the free stuff she'd get. Hysterically, she'd ask them if they had items in low fat or reduced calorie versions. As though Joyce was at a local store! Then, her old time recipes were given makeovers that left them still tasty but healthier. She'd followed my suggestions that there were more condiments than butter, ketchup and ranch dressing. Like a kid at Christmas, each new spice, vinegar, healthy oil or seasoning was greeted with wide eyed wonder and enthusiasm at its very existence. You could feel the fun at Joyce's slim parade.

Well, the only downside I really heard Joyce say was that her husband was getting jealous and possessive of her now that she was looking so good. Remember, she was still wearing her seemingly endless supply of Flashdance style torn shirts over spandex. Now, at her heaviest, this was not bothering her spouse. But, now that she was nearing 149# (a milestone figure. Joyce hadn't been under 150 since Junior High) the old man was unhappy that her 'fine ass was on display for any guy to look at', to quote directly. Well, if Joyce had to have a problem that could be it, right?

When Joyce made goal, she cried with joy. Her before and after shots were mouth dropping examples of what she was capable of. She looked at least 20 years younger. Dressing in young style clothes were never a problem for Joyce. The transformation was primarily of her profound pride in what she'd done. No one had faith in her that she'd stick with it. Her sisters, husband, friends all continued their unhealthy overeating ways and Joyce plowed right through all the potential obstacles like they weren't even there. I think that for her they weren't.

TIPS: Be open to new foods! I only know one thing about every new person when we meet - they need to change their eating habits. Joyce rocked this from day one and her loss sped up a lot because of it. New foods = new treasures.

TRAPS: Only impending catastrophe brought Joyce to her senses. Will you remain a sedentary overweight smoker that's determined to ignore all until you pay seriously high health prices? Don't!

HOW LONG IS THIS GONNA TAKE?:

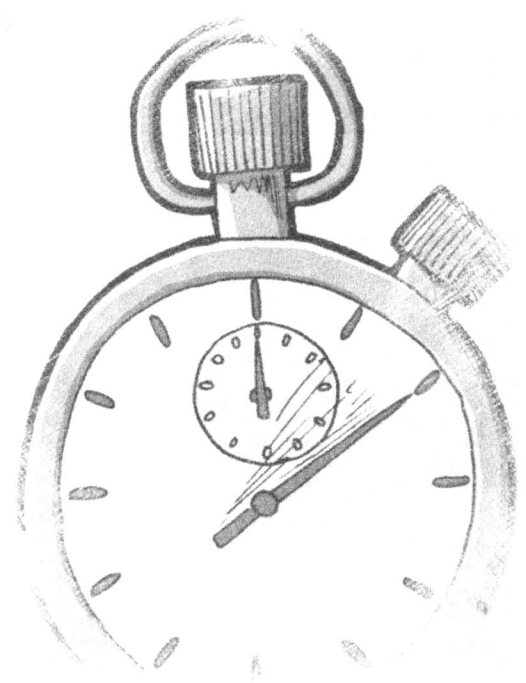

I was greeting members in a hoppin' busy weigh in session when I saw her. A tiny old lady dressed like a hip hopper. Not 5' tall, with a tangerine tint in her hair (or at least a tangerine weave), bell flared jeans, jean jacket (both with studs), a funky denim hat turned sideways, chunky gold costume jewelry dangling from many places and bright gold sneakers on her tiny feet. Make up caked all over her wrinkled face. She looked like a caricature from a comedy sketch show. More to the point, yes, her attire made her stand out, but there was more to her. She just stood in the doorway like she expected someone to walk over and explain what she was doing there to her. I obliged. All the way across the room I was also wondering what this woman was doing there. Not only was she dressed like one of the Beastie Boys' grandmother, but she was skinny as a stick. I'm sure she didn't weigh 100#. I introduced myself, she looked up (a lifelong necessity, I'm sure) and asked me 'How long is this gonna take?'

I was alternately amused and surprised. Amused by her voice - an old lady whine I've also heard in many a comedy show skit (think New Yorker in Miami) and amazed by her question. How long is this gonna take? I surprised myself when the perfect retort came naturally out of my mouth. I said, 'The rest of your life.' I usually hesitate and regroup my mind when people ask me crazy things. It's an asset, I've found. When people are rude, it happens, too: again, an asset. I don't shoot my mouth off immediately and say something I'll regret or will get me in trouble later. So, when this entirely logical, non-confrontational, simply perfect answer calmly came out of my mouth, I was impressed and grateful.

Now, for the little lady's reaction: 'Oh', echoed with great disappointment. It was right then and there that I decided I liked her. She didn't get offended or argue with the truth of my answer. Some people don't like being told the truth, especially in regards to their food life. She seemed to understand what I'd said and seemed to accept it. I told her of the prices, the basic overview of the program and mentioned that she may not qualify for membership because she was too skinny. Yes, there is such a thing as being too thin. The program requires a minimum of 5# be lost to join. I've had an occasional person be turned away for that reason. Sufferers of anorexia or bulimia are not allowed. We cannot help them.

It seemed she accepted that it was a lifestyle change. She was just looking for a diet to lose a few pounds, really. I told her that that was just fine and that the program was not for everybody and that she maybe didn't need to sign up for this. She gave me a funny, 'oh, what the hell' shrug and decided to proceed. I was surprised she was just 5# over the minimum weight for her height. I have a feeling it was bogus since she weighed in wearing jeans and sneakers (Lord, those gold sneakers!) I see them on the stylish elderly all the time now. She was my first. Little did I know she was ahead of her time setting a trend: Lady Gaga, Sr. Out she went with the material probably to a hip hop concert or vintage clothing exchange store.

Well, week two comes and she walks in, made a bee line for me and speaks up about her confusion over this or that. Also trying to bargain with good health suggestions we make. I'm used to members trying to get out of what they don't want to do. Heck, I'm a master at that. I wrote the playbook on it. Gaga, Sr. seemed again to take my answers well. She moped a bit, but never disagreed. I was trying to be diplomatic and logical in all my replies No wit or irony or over talking would do with this case. Being relatable is the key to getting members to trust you and open up about their needs. She weighed in, lost a bit and sat down. I'd told her not to expect a big drop. At her weight and age, it would not be realistic. I only got semi stern with her on one thing - no gimmicky diet nonsense. That was what she'd come in the door looking for and had spent her entire life dabbling in. Magic shakes, bars, mix-ins, smoothies, rice cakes, vitamins and sprinkles that are as phony as a Milli Vanilli record.

After a few weeks, she came up to me and told me she would not be coming back. It wasn't for her. She wasn't like most of these people that were so fat (her exact words). Despite the slight insult in her choice of words, I know she didn't mean it in malice. I agreed it truly wasn't for her. We smiled and I wished her well. Then, I turned my attention to these poor unfortunate creatures she'd graciously released me from her to unburden.

"How long is this gonna take?" is a very common question members ask. Speed isn't emphasized in the program. In fact, if anything, it's de-emphasized. Everyone who joins has been overweight for XX amount of years, but now wants it all off in a flash. Who doesn't, right? But I stand by my answer to this day: 'For the rest of your life'. Or to translate it to more hands on terms for the immediate needs of new members, 'Well, that's up to you. The more closely you follow the program the quicker it'll be. But, I'm not clocking you.'

Bottom line: the same amount of time will pass weather you do this or if you don't. If I could look into a crystal ball and tell someone a precise time, such as, 'It'll take 2 and 1/2 years'. If their reaction would be, 'Oh, that's WAY too slow. I'm gonna go find something else', I'd say as they were leaving, 'You're making a mistake!' I know the program works better than any other out there. I know it. So, I love to propose that anyone can be thin in 2 and 1/2 years' time or they can be heavy or heavier than they are now still spinning their wheels. Either way, the same amount of time will pass. It's up to them, but I am not objective about trying to persuade them of the wisdom of the latter option.

One more time: "How long is this gonna take?" - Permanent lifestyle changes don't come with guarantees, schedules or deadlines. If you see it that way, it makes it easier.

TIPS: If anything surprised me regarding this lady, it was how well she took the truth when it was said to her. How receptive are you to it? You can't bargain with biology.

TRAPS: Her traps are the ones we often fall for: looking for magic, speed fixes. Who doesn't want them? If you believe they're out there, you won't apply yourself to any long term, real world sensible program. Also, being too thin can be a trap. Yes, it IS possible.

ZACK AND ANNE:

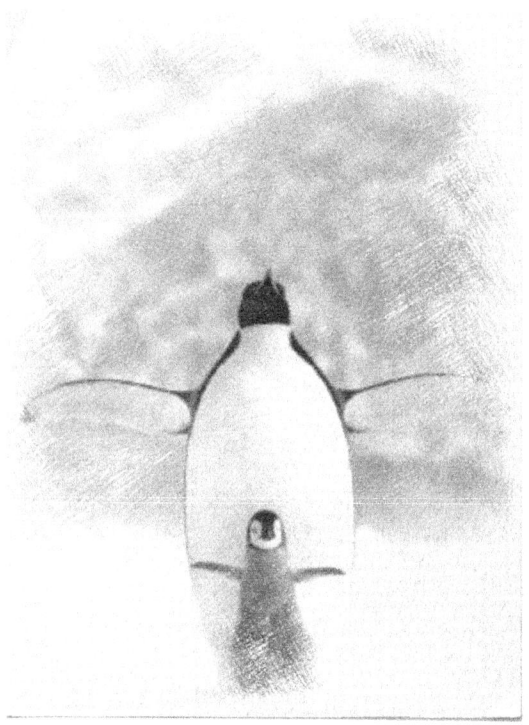

I have a profile in this series regarding kids. The four stories were kids I didn't see on a consistent basis and were very damaged young people. I regrettably didn't see recovery in any of them. Their wounds and needs were too long and deep to be remotely satisfied solely by me. Their parents were just kidding themselves or lazily pawning off the problem. I can't say.

Zack was different. Primarily for two reasons: though a teen of 15 or so when I first met him and a serious 60+# overweight, I would have his presence in the rooms for the duration this would take. This was done by his awesome and caring fellow member mother, Anne. She was an example of the proper parental role in supportive co-piloting a teen through this. The other reason, Zack was obviously very intelligent and mature beyond his years. Not shy, well-spoken and keenly aware of why he was there. Zack needed his mother's assistance in only the ways any parent would need to be. She drove them to the meetings, she paid, she shopped thoughtfully, she was aware of the program so he wouldn't be expected to navigate alone at 15. What a pair!

As I got to know Zack, not much really surprised me. He was an honor student. He was very into technology. He was not happy being overweight and intended to use his skillful ways of studying to his advantage here. Just like in school. As I've said before, I can tell easily when members are 'there in body only' or 'there in body, mind and spirit.' Zack was all there —very present. He shared wise experiences in class and he seemed disturbed by the horrible nutrition conditions in his school. I told him it was a national epidemic that he was being made aware of. He brought lunches. He shared an interest in the grocery shopping. He, his mother and their calculator made thorough trips down supermarket aisles pondering the wisest choices. When it was especially good, they'd let us know.

I brought up if the father was also supportive. I pitied daddy if he wasn't. This was no passive duo that would be stifled by anyone. He was, they assured me. Good —I never mentioned it again. If anything, as an overachiever, Zack began to eclipse his mother. She was a lifetime member, looked smashing at goal but fell into the too,

too common trap of relaxing her discipline, letting her weekly class attendance lapse, predictably put on pounds and not want to come back and pay......I remain endlessly baffled when members tell me this. A few solo attempts to come back and reignite the fire were not successful for Anne. Eventually, she had all her 50+# on again.

Enter Zack. He kept her accountable and the child became the parent. I'm glad to say the balance of support seemed stable throughout all of this. I have watched WAY too many duos implode when one does much better than the other. This has happened with parent / child, friends, siblings, husband / wife, boyfriend / girlfriend, co-work-ers.... the worst cases are when the one doing better is dragged down by the other: such a shame.

Anne came weekly with Zack, not really 'in the game'. I could tell, admired her unforced admiration for her son and offered her any private extra time, support, track review or whatever she may need to reconnect. She thanked me although she never took me up on the offer. "I just have to get my mind around the fact that it has to be a permanent lifestyle change. I thought I was gonna be an exception, I really did. I could just splurge occasionally and get away with it. Or track in my head…I learned the hard way I'm not an exception. I'm just like everybody else."...me, too. I embrace this. It makes it much easier.

Anne took inspiration from her son and at long last surrendered her resistance and re applied herself to the program with the orig-inal fierce determination she'd had when she made goal originally. The 50+ extra pounds she was carrying went away again. This time she's making good on her vow to continue to be the diligent member she is and keep it off by keeping strong, focused, attending classes and knowing that it's for life. Good for Anne, she deserves it and looks amazing.

Zack made goal with a 50+# weight loss. He'd made it look easy and celebrated being 16 with both a slim body and a driver's license. What a kid. Unlike this writer's flaky on and off adolescent commitment level, Zack stayed his freckle faced serious self about maintenance. He seemed to get it...on the first shot ... as a KID! Only school kept him away. Now, in college, he's studying to do something computer/software design related. You can see, I'm not a techy person at all. One day he'll probably be a billionaire. Remember the humble folks that helped you when you were young, I've told him jokingly. He assured me that he will.

My final and happiest thought about Zack is the life he'll lead as an adult: How much crap he won't endure. The distractions being in the grips of food obsession is. The self-esteem battering that occurs. The socializing you don't do. Settling for "less than" friends or girl-friends; leisure activities that are all affected by being as heavy as he was. Career limitations when people pre judge you negatively for being overweight. Yes, we know that exists. The calmer, happier life Zack will have not dodging icebergs. All this will be Zack's. He may not fully realize how much grief he's spared himself, but I know. His mother certainly knows.

TIPS: Be an amazingly exceptional teen! I know that's not possible for the majority or it wouldn't be called amazing. It would be called average. If you're in a duo and you're doing the better of the two, reach out and try to elevate your partner.

TRAPS: But if they refuse, don't let it overtake you. Zack was very strong and his mother did come to model him. As the lesser accomplished of a duo, never throw mud, mope, apply guilt or try to discourage your partner in any way. Don't damage their chance.

TINA:

When people join the program, they're very wounded. Broken bodies, spirits, hopes and promises are the clay I am given to work with. I am in my element. I have been that person. It takes a great deal of courage to walk into a class room. Admitting you have a problem you cannot manage yourself is very difficult for many. It's my desire and privilege to try to mold them into people who are able to achieve things they didn't think possible.

Part of this process involves winning the trust of members. Some walk in already knowing the program works. Some require convincing. The magic of the class experience and other members is the water that allows the clay to be reformed at this particular chapter of the journey. I don't hold back in my classes. I admit my flaws, embarrassing situations and compulsions and relapses freely. It helps members lower their defenses and see what I've been through is often close to what they're dealing with. I understand and have overcome many demons right where they are sitting.

I'm known for my very candid, blunt confessions. A member who hears their own shameful behavior discussed in front of them has a way of winning them over. It's common for overweight people to hold onto great amounts of shame. We carry it around and its ponderous weight drags us further into a cycle of negative self-images. Knowing they're surrounded by people who have also eaten in the dark of a basement or closet, gobbled down fast food meals in the car and thrown the evidence out the window, rearranged cookie displays in a church bake sale, snuck treats in any manner of ways that would confound Sherlock Holmes has a way of bonding folks.

Classic story: On my way to join the program, I ate two cherry Hostess fruit pies —in the car. I was shoving them in literally on the way there. Like an alcoholic drinking a bottle of whiskey on their way to rehab. I lived tragically close to the center so I arrived far too quickly for the consumption of my latest 'last binge'. I took the last 1/3rd of my pastry and inhaled it. Then, you know that you ate too big a bite, didn't chew it well enough, then swallowed it and semi choked feeling? That's how I walked in the door. Rubbing the remnants of greasy sugar off my face, coughing, gagging - "Uh, I'm here ... to.... join. Or drop dead, whichever comes first." Members love that one.

In my candid confession mode, I told the story of how you can learn to lie and manipulate people at a very, very young age. In the name of food, I was in a constant search for more. I was already practicing my methods of sneaking, fibbing, rearranging the ice creams, peanut butter and other goodies thinking I would not be found out ... it was an ongoing endeavor.

As I'd said in my disclosure, I would lie to my mother, saying that I had to go to the bathroom when we were in the supermarket. Then, I'd run to the baking isle, grab tubes of icing, unscrew the cap and squeeeeeeze it into my mouth. As much goopy sugary delightful icing as I dared. Screw the cap back on, hang it back up, gulp it down as quickly as I could and meet my mother again. Probably with an unnatural colored tongue from what flavor I'd inhaled. I never buy those things to this day. Someone else must have done that, too.

Fast forward to a member's successful journey to goal: her name was Tina. She was a tall, blonde, beautiful lady who lost over 40 pounds to transform into a woman with an envy inducing figure, lovely face and personality that would make doors open for her anyplace. Also, with a small daughter in tow, she would be a glorious example for her.

A few weeks after goal, she gave me a card. When members give me the honor of sharing personal thoughts, I read them privately. I am an easy cry, and I have to keep my composure. Well, in her letter, she said that in her youth she, too, had lied about bathroom trips she didn't need to take and snuck icing from the tubes. She'd never told a single soul. She'd never heard anyone ever say it. She wrote that when I told my own story about that, she nearly fell out of her chair. Her continued success on the program seems very likely. She is taking exercise classes because she knows food discipline is only half of it. Activity plays a crucial part, too. Her words moved me deeply. The shame whirlpool we take ourselves down can consume us. Releasing the shackles of the past allows us to metamorphosis into the true selves some of us had never met.

Tina is not only a glorious lady, but a reminder of how much being brutally honest is for me and will always be a key part of my classes. I will always be the first one to admit to eating food out of my kitchen garbage, following the 5 second rule with something I've dropped on the floor, pretending I'm ordering 2 burgers and 2 fries for 2 people by ordering 2 beverages.... you get the idea. It makes me relatable. It frees members to unburden themselves. It can make us laugh, sometimes. It heals.

TIPS: You won't be young forever. Tina exercises because she knows food discipline alone won't keep her slim. It'd take too much restriction for that. Do you intend to rely on 100% diet perfection? It's not very possible and completely unnecessary.

TRAPS: Holding on to shame is like mold. It festers, grows and causes much damage that can wreck the sturdiest foundation. Most overweight people have done all kinds of wacky, desperate and embarrassing things. You're much more 'normal' than you know. ½ of everyone around you has done it, too. Release your shame!

YVONNE AND JOE:

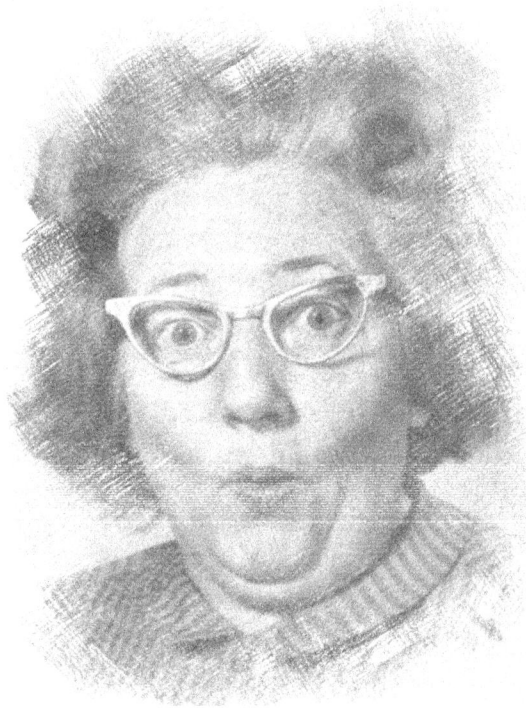

Yvonne was frustrated. I weighed her and she didn't get the results she was after. Her chagrined expression was echoed by my desire to help her. It's one of the great fulfilling aspects of my job. I love to help people succeed. It's my passion. It significantly altered my life, truth be told. I certainly allowed other branches of a balanced life fall to the wayside. Being fixated on one cause seems to be my strong suit. Multi-tasking is not.

But I digress, back to Yvonne. I know her type: the 'Ida Know' lady. Joins, is pleasant, shares in class; seems to be listening. But, in the results department— lacks. Weeks go by and my advice seems to be adhered to and my hopes rise for her only to be dashed the next week after another disappointing weigh in. The excuse rolodex comes out and we spin the wheel. I know the excuse rolodex well, too. I've used it. I've written a few volumes. I've relied on it to justify my behavior. Makes indulging less guilt inducing.

Guilt mucks up digestion. I told so many of my teachers excuse after excuse. They'd patiently hear me and nod their head and I'd sit down for the class and begin sulking. I wonder if they were thinking to themselves the same things I think when I'm given recitations from the latest addition to the international excuse rolodex. "Sheesh, this guy's hopeless! How much I'd love to just tell him exactly what I think - NO, what I KNOW - is the reality of his situation. But, I can't."

Of course, they did. I think it often. But I digress, yet again. This is not typical of me. It's difficult for this blunt talker to silently hear excuses that I know are just that. Yvonne had been thin in her younger years and gained weight as years passed but was not willing to fully embrace what was required of her to lose weight. Her company was pleasant. Her smile was sincere. Her friends were equally unsuccessful in their half-hearted going through the motions time in my class. That was also doing Yvonne no good at all. Excuse makers LOVE like- minded company. They resist challenges and resent the good intentions behind them. They're buzz kills. Ewwww, eat less - move more - no using worn out phrases that lost any semblance of meaning but seem to appease. Not wanted!

So, why was I surprised that she didn't take my advice, my GREAT advice with open arms and an open mind? I am very good at assessing individual's mind set to customize my approach. There is no 'one solution suits all'. HA! How convenient that would be. Alas, the slower, more labor intensive way is the right way. Why is that so often the case? Mother Nature is a funny lady!

Her husband's name was Joe. I know this because she spoke of him constantly. I never met Joe. Joe doesn't join diet groups. That's for women. I have heard that song sung by MANY women who've lamented their husbands, boyfriends, father's weight problems. "Oh, but he'd NEVER join." Implication: It's not a manly thing to do. Men don't need help. They probably pull their punches simply because I am a man and they don't wish to offend. Well, at least I hope that's why. I DO try to think the best of people. Joe was an unsupportive fella. He needed his meat and potatoes every night. He needed bread and butter. He needed his favorite cake and casserole ...I will never know how much Joe was being used as a scapegoat. It's possible Joe was a perfectly agreeable type who would have gladly adjusted to healthier eating. Perhaps Joe was the ogre Yvonne described. Well, there are ways around both. One doesn't exist in a bubble. Your surroundings have a large impact on what your daily struggle level is. I know this. My own family was level medium on that. Joe evidently was nil.

"Joe is wrong." Wow, I said it, finally! One night, after another no weight loss weigh in, Yvonne threatened quitting in frustration yet again. "Joe said this and Joe said that" about why she's wasting her money or there's no way she can expect to lose weight on this program and blah, blah, blah. With no more desire to do my part in this charade, I looked Yvonne in the eye and said "Joe is wrong." She got goggle eyed, was struck dumb, stepped back and looked at me as though I'd said "God is wrong." She just sat down. Sigh. I know I will not reach her. She is beyond my help, maybe beyond anyone's help. Thankfully, her type of woman is not the norm any longer. It's partly generational. It's from another time: women acquiesced decision making process to men, leaving their sphere to solely 'female areas'; cooking, cleaning, child rearing (in certain areas), sewing... Reared from the start that their rightful place is to trust and obey in a child-like manner for too many decades has left Yvonne like many other women: senior citizen body and an undeveloped mind for most of life's problems. When I said, "Joe is wrong" she simply didn't know what to say. If Joe is wrong, then she'd have no basis for living as her own devices were rusty, perhaps beyond cranking up to usability. Joe has filled Yvonne with a lot of nonsense that's permeated into her too deeply, for too long, for an outsider to penetrate in a matter of months.

Unsurprisingly, Yvonne didn't stick around after that, never to be seen by me again. I would love nothing better than to be wrong, but I probably am not. Maybe she tried other nonsense diets that TV personalities offered. Her friends in her small circle exchanged half-baked ideas. I'll never know. If she's still living, she's quite advanced in years now. If she's passed, she was a nice lady and I enjoyed her company. Her type of upbringing has diminished with successive generations of women, making Yvonnes less common. I have a great love of seniors. I have managed to crack the old code with many of them and seen them accomplish weight loss after many, even themselves, had given up. I continue to see all members, seniors included, with 100% belief that they can take charge of their life, weight and therefore destiny. I always will. The Yvonnes that never rise above the ditch they'd been put into virtually from birth are part of my fire I draw from.

TIPS: To be fair, I can't know if all Yvonne said about Joe is true. Don't fib to your teachers, it's not necessary. Also, very likely it's not believed. Do you have a circle of friends who nurture denial or off putting blame? They're toxic. Move on. Honesty brings success.

TRAPS: Passing your life decisions off on another for ANY reason leaves you a child with 'victim' written all over you. Take charge of your own life and destiny.

MISTY:

"WOOOO, SIX KIDS and A SIZE SIX!!!" I can bet they're still talking about this at the store where Misty shouted those words from the dressing room. Trying on form fitting slacks, at her goal weight size, she was celebrating reaching goal via the program the right way - not with food! Her transformation came against all the accepted reasons women in her situation allow to take on a role they should not. As a mother, a woman over 35, a wife, a community oriented - church going - charity volunteering - little league driving - all around great lady of suburbia. I meet this type of woman in the program so often I should consider them job security. In their stretch pants or mom jeans, often these women are far too young for their attire and the ailments it has brought, as was Misty, but she was ready to change.

It cannot be overstated how much this mind set is a pre requisite to success in the program. Actually, I think it's a pre requisite to just about any endeavor you may want to undertake. If it isn't in your head to be fully engaged, the odds are very small that you'll accomplish much of anything. This is very true for weight loss. Misty had played by the rules all her life. Blond, pretty, friendly, giving, easy to talk to and obviously a woman who'd made family her top priority - Misty had let her own health and weight become a lower and lower concern until it became a problem she was unwilling to ignore longer.

Six kids will certainly take your focus and energy. I recall a co-worker of mine from my past who also had six kids. I used to ask her how she managed, particularly when they were all small. She said she just didn't do ANYthing else but cook, clean, do laundry, iron, take them wherever they needed to be .... for at least a decade. When she looked up, she found a big gap in her knowledge of what was going on in the world. She'd often say that 1969 to 1980 references to politics, pop culture, trends, hit songs, fads or famous news items were all missed. By the way, this overweight lady also joined the program at my class. I was very proud of her.

Misty was at a point where the youngest one was in school and she was experiencing, if not empty nest quite yet, at least some time on her hands after that decade of blurry chaos that I'd just described. Misty assessed herself. She was not happy with her weight. 50 extra pounds on a 5'4" frame was not flattering and she was truly 'seeing it' for the first time in many years. She knew too many other women in her same dynamic that had just accepted the extra weight. She

2345678910111213

was not going to. She was 45, not 70! Wisely, Misty had her husband watch the kids. The classes are not social events. She'd taken time out of a very busy schedule to learn what she needed to do to get thin. She'd put her valuable time and trust into the program and as a conveyor of that program - into me, as well. I was determined to deliver. I knew she could do this!

With a relaxed demeanor some people don't see the steely determined game plan that's underneath the surface. I knew Misty was working the program. She asked questions in class. This is very, very wise. I come across too many people who are tight lipped when I offer Q and A at the start of all classes. The class is the most fertile soil to plant seeds in and nurture. Why every hand isn't up baffles me week after week. Suffering people that sit there hoping someone else will ask what they want to know are wasting their time, money and allowing their motivation to dim as they squander this chance. It's one thing to not speak up in social occasions, but they're PAYING for this. I just don't get it. Misty was going to get what she'd come there for.

Misty was enjoying getting slim so much, I was as eager to hear her victories as the members were. She was so overjoyed with her shrinking body that she couldn't contain her enthusiasm. Why should she? This was one dynamic woman accomplishing what she'd put aside for the sake of her children for over 15 years and bucked conventional thinking that it shouldn't be something to aspire to 'at her age'. The big payoff is in the increased energy, improved self-esteem, less pain, different relationships based on respect and, of course, CLOTHES!!

Being overweight makes clothes shopping miserable. Misty had had it with drab, formless clothes that made up most of her wardrobe.

She and I connected on many levels. One of the big ones being we were both clothes obsessed. Too many years on the outside looking in at stylish, attractive clothes had left both of us with a burning desire to breakthrough this glass and take full advantage of going into any store and buying whatever you want. This is a big reward for not eating the way we used to. It's one of the best ones. I didn't give up eating peanut butter and ice cream....in gargantuan amounts daily to NOT wear flattering clothes. Misty, too, was not going to take off all this weight and dress in gray, beige, black or navy blue dull, drab, cheap unflattering garments. No way.

Misty gained weight a few times. We all have to go up to bat and strike out sometimes. It makes us human. She never made excuses for it and never avoided classes because she'd wanted to bury her head in the sand. That never works. She'd own it, purge it and move on. THAT is how members make goal. It's not people who never stumble - that's normal. It's those who know how to pick themselves up, dust themselves off and get back up on the horse and keep riding. Misty had that quality big time!

Wearing white after Labor Day appeals to me not only because I am a firm believer in not obeying sensible fashion rules, but also because it represents something. White is the least slimming color one can wear. I mention often in my classes that one of my ultimate clothes dreams I'd harbored was being able to wear pure white jeans in my goal weight size. When it happened, I put them on in the dressing room and checked myself out mercilessly from every angle I could get at in the 3- way mirror. Front, back, bending over, squatting, dancing ... all those things we can only do in the safety of a dressing room. When I realized I looked alright, I stood there and took the moment in. I said out loud, 'You've waited 20 years for this.'

Misty did what I should have done. She, too, evidently was a big fan of white. She got a pair of non-stretch contour cut white jeans to her dressing room. When they fit, she didn't take in the moment quietly. She put her fists in the air and shouted, "SIX KIDS and A SIZE SIX!!!" That's how I want all of my members to celebrate goal: loud, proud and jubilantly. Misty will be the foxiest grandmother in town, too!

TIPS: Let clothes be a fire for you. Whatever you're looking at on others or in magazines, old photos of you - buy them again. They're tremendously motivating.

TRAPS: Don't buy into 'mom thinking': Mothers who bury themselves in the rearing of kids to the extent that their own well-being suffers. It isn't easy, but the two are not mutually exclusive.

OPAL AND LAURA:

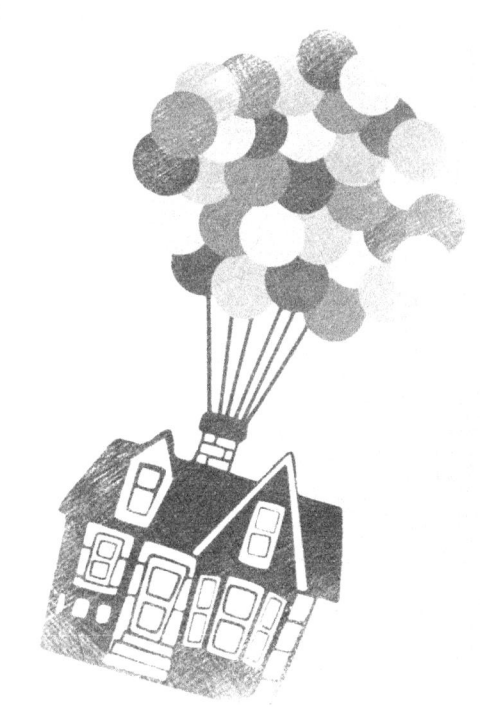

Mother / daughter duos joining the program aren't uncommon. Women are much more willing to join groups than men seem to be. This is one of the arguments for women being smarter! Also, a network of family support is always very useful: "Talking the same language", "On the same page" and all that. So, when Opal and Laura joined, it was part of what they hoped would work to their advantage. Laura, the daughter, looked 50 something, and well put together.

Cool haircut, well thought out accessories, fashionable shoes, make up not overdone but obviously care put into it. This type of over-weight woman tells a story. She still cares about her appearance enough to put in time and effort. Laura was 70 or so pounds over-weight. What she had in style she lacked in drive, sadly. A successful businesswoman, she offered all the cliché excuses - busy, stressed, travels, doesn't cook, can't exercise because of this limitation or that one .... blah, blah, blah.

Opal, the mother, was a pistol. Short, sassy and senior. She was 50 pounds or so overweight, and on her smaller frame, it looked like more. Laura must have a tall father. Like many older people with that much extra poundage, she was always complaining about her fatigue, bad back, tired legs, sore joints and all the baggage that time and fat exacerbates. She was blunt in that 'I'm old and don't care what anyone thinks' way that I find appealing. I am that way, too. But, I'm still in my working years and it's gotten me in trouble more than once. A perk of being old that I'm looking forward to is when no one cares about what I say or think enough to be offended.

I didn't have a lot of hope for them, but we clicked and the weight slowly came off. Laura really did travel a lot and missed many classes because of that. This never helps. Also, her schedule required that she see different teachers on different days in different locations. "Hoppers", we call 'em. They rarely do well. Opal didn't drive and was at Laura's mercy regarding this. It frustrated her and was interfer-ing with her progress. After a few good old fashioned chats, we con-vinced Laura of the necessity and value of consistency and she began following me to any location I was at, Opal, in tow. Good move!

Laura lost some weight, but never got 100% into a groove. Never less than well-groomed with her latest reason why it didn't happen. Food in Tokyo hotels are impossible to even identify, let alone assess. Hmmm, what can I say to that?

On the other hand, Opal blossomed: lost weight, gained mobility, spoke frankly but with positive twists that made very valuable points whenever she spoke, which was at most classes. Her posture improved and some of Laura's style rubbed off. She began showing up in glitter jackets, make up on (too much, but I don't know how her eyesight was), chic black slacks and a smile that spoke as loudly as 100 speakers. She'd never been this thin in her entire life. There was no stopping her and who'd want to? Making goal was her happy ending. She was ecstatic and unlocked a key in her head to commit to health that she knew she'd keep her entire life. Her only regret, she hadn't made the switch sooner. She tried to credit me with the transformation, but I deflected it back to her, knowing she had slayed the beast.

Attendance remained sporadic due to Laura's travels. So, it was not too much concern for me when they were not there. Laura quit and rejoined over and over again for a few years. I never make re- joiners feel any criticism or judged when they walk back in. That was my path, too. I know how lousy they feel and only want them to see the possibility that this is the time they'll get it together. After all, Opal was over 75 and she'd done it; it's never too late! Not until you take you final breath.

Laura was alone when I had her last rejoin (she would never return after this). She said Opal had passed away peacefully with loved ones around her. After hugs, she said that being thin at her life's end was the final accomplishment she needed to do. It had reinvigorated her zest for living and made her last years truly golden. She had asked to be buried in one of those stylish outfits she'd proudly strutted into her classes wearing: a slim angel. I'll never forget her.

TIPS: Consistency helps! The same counselor, weigh day, meeting time all allow you to make bonds, develop accountability, rapport and more accurate gauges of your body's rhythm and progress.

TRAPS: Laura's keeping up all other aspects of her appearance. While it's very commendable, it's not a substitute for weight loss. As for the common age trap, Opal didn't fall for that!

ADAM:

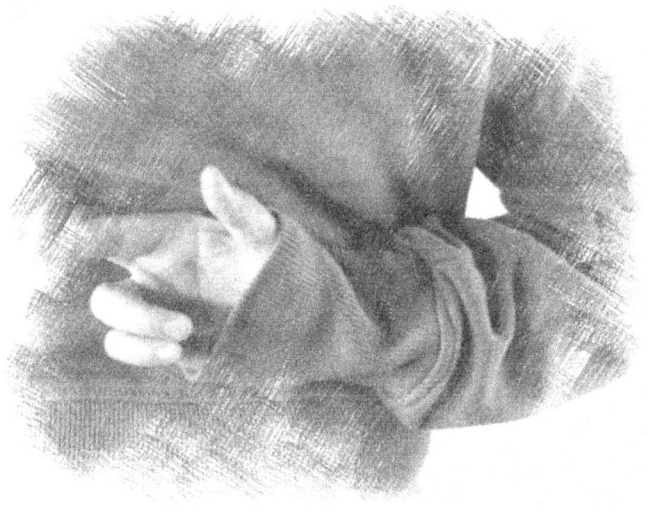

Adam. A nice fellow I met when I was teaching a class in a small town on the Nevada / Utah border. We met in the rec center: sort of a mini YMCA. I was stared at every week as I walked through the place like a visiting Martian. I dress in flashy clothes. It's one of my trademarks. My members enjoy it, it makes me smile and as a marketing strategy, it's paid off. Also, bright colors improve the mood. They loved me in the other small town I'd taught at. This one was not overly friendly to me. Still...head held high, I have learned to ignore the haters. At least I put on a brave face. I'm very thin skinned, to be honest. More than I should be at my age.

Adam was a 20 something man involved in scouting: a very big enterprise in their community. He needed to lose weight because he was simply too heavy to take the troops on the vigorous hiking, swimming, camping, walking type of endeavors that are typical of the scouts. He'd been given the ultimatum of 'lose weight or lose your post'. His mother was already a member of the program so he followed her there.

Now, armed with personal motivation that he took seriously, Adam was a model member. He lost weight weekly and rapidly ... too rapidly, to be honest. But he spoke engagingly at meetings, had ties to the fellow members and was pleasant to have around. Small towns often have a tight network of socializing. They often all seemed to know the same places restaurants, holiday rituals.... I admit I got fooled by him. I thought at his young age, goal was both possible and inevitable.

Suddenly, he was gone. I saw his mother weekly and asked where he was and she often mumbled reasons that didn't ring sincere. Bad liar, she was. Maybe that's a good thing. As I've said, people lie in classes a lot. So, I was deflated by his disappearing act. After a few weeks, I stopped asking. Then, the truth came out on its own. Adam was only there to get to the very border of the weight maximum for scouting and bolted the minute his weight record showed it. He never intended to see it through.

But, as often happens when ulterior motives are disingenuous, it bit Adam back big time. He went on an eating bender that so alarmed his mother that she finally told me what I'd already deciphered. He was gorging on food and visibly regained an alarming amount of weight in a very short time. His mother was worried about him inducing a heart attack. Adam didn't think it through. Sure, his class record had the number he was at the last attendance. But, he didn't expect the scouts would require more. When you got to the doctor's office for a physical, they WEIGH you! They don't take the written document from another source! It's the same with the scouts. Adam was not allowed to do what he loved with his spare time, to nurture future Eagle Scouts because he was both a poor fitness example and a liability simply because he was not likely able to participate in the leisure or official physical activities.

Moral - honesty is always best. I would have understood and prepared him for a better route to keep weight off and work on the attitude for a permanent lifestyle change required to make him healthy enough to be a Scouting coach for many years. Excuses claim another casualty.

TIPS: Adam wanted to lead a troop of Scouts. There are requirements to be suited for it. That got Adam in the door. A great reason to start is usually personal. However, ...

TRAPS: When events are your sole motivation, it often leads to temporary success. A high school reunion, vacations - they're all great first mountains to climb toward. But, I guarantee you, those occasions come and then they go! When all your eggs are in one basket, your motivation can disappear too easily.

CLAIRE:

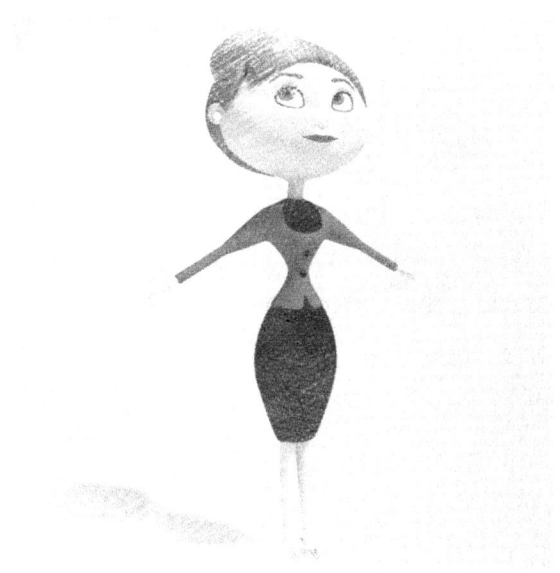

"My husband wants me to get back to my high school weight". I stood and stared at the 60+ year old, tiny lady looking up at me with a matter of fact expression on her face. She was a potential joiner. She was petite, not too overweight, had longer hair than is common for women her age (I love when any woman bucks any trend towards not shining in any way she could 'because of her age'). She didn't seem to think this was an unreasonable thing for her husband to expect. Not disrespectful or unkind, unforgiving, unfair or any other 'un' you'd care to add.

Sometimes, when I meet someone in my capacity, someone says something outrageous and I organically come up with the perfect retort on the spot. This doesn't always happen. Often, I'm struck dumb and think of the best answer later, but, not this day. I looked right down at her raccoon mascara eyes and said, "Well, is he at HIS high school weight?"

Oh, snap, I was glad I'd said that. Claire stared at me in disbelief. Oh, another one of these ladies, I thought to myself. The generation of women like Claire that were inducted into this type of thinking has been replaced by more independent, confident women conducting more fulfilling lives. Claire laughed with me at the thought. I was glad she'd taken it with good humor. It was a deciding moment in our potential working relationship. If she was going to succeed on the program, she'd have to come into her own. Good for you, Claire.

In her upbringing, men were allowed full release from any concern about their appearance. They could get obese, bald, wrinkled as leather, dress like bums, ignore their hygiene and still if they provided a paycheck or had a pulse, depending on just how desperate one was, it didn't matter. Women were expected to keep their figure as this was their role in this double standard ridiculous game. Women still bear the short end of this arrangement to this day. Has it improved? Yes. Does it still exist? Sadly, yes.

Claire had bought into the entire bag of goods many years ago. She was pleasant, upbeat, dressed young and kinda quirky: in other words, my kind of lady. Her mind must have had a thirst she wasn't fully aware existed until she joined the program. 'Is my husband at his high school weight?' Claire pondered this comment a lot. It seemed he wasn't. It seemed he was overweight and hadn't seen his high school weight since perhaps when Chubby Checker was doing the twist. Funny as it was, there was a creepy undercurrent to Claire's obedient entrance into a 'diet club' at his command that she return, at over 60, to a weight she'd been as a teenager.

I decided not to focus on this as it was Claire that I wanted to see lose weight for herself, and herself alone. The health benefits and increase in her own self-worth were at stake here and I felt like I didn't want to rock the boat too early in her time here or she might quit. High self-esteem often means sassing back at overbearing people in one's life that have had it coming for too long.

Claire would grow in confidence as her body shrunk.

Honestly, she'd missed her calling as a professional comedienne. Like Gracie Allen or Edith Bunker, part of her funny nature was her delivery was totally as if what she said wasn't funny at all. I looked forward to seeing her every week in some garish bright workout outfit on that the 8Os didn't destroy. Her commitment to getting healthy was genuine, no matter the impetus. She loved to exercise. That's not the common thing with my members. The US surgeon general regularly delivers grim stats on how much of the US adult population is inactive to fully sedentary. Claire was a firecracker.

Bless her heart, she'd share excited stories about reading romance novels and wishing her husband was 1/2 the lover the fictional Fabio styled fantasy was. How spinach gave her gas. Her husband's chronic bad breath inspired her to put mouthwash in his iced tea. Hysterical! All the time the class would erupt in laughter, she'd just wait for it to die down without the slightest expression that she said anything funny. How could her husband not adore this lady just as she was? I didn't get it. Not my business.

Since Claire was firing at her weight problem from both guns from day one - steady activity plus now a sensible food program, the pounds came off steadily. One again, a senior silver star that disproves the notion that people over a certain age cannot lose weight - nonsense! They will just naturally get heavy and there's nothing that can be done - untrue! Yes, Claire got back to her high school weight. We were all so happy for her. But I held back a small black thought because I didn't want to take any wind out of her sails. It ticked me off that her husband got what he wanted. It was a chauvinistic, out of line request he'd given her. She should have told him to get lost. But, for her sake, I never broached it.

Claire is now in her late 70s, still slim, still active, still dressing in bright tacky clothes, happy and oblivious to anyone trying to bring her down. I hope I'm like her when I'm that age. Claire, you rock!

TIPS: Activity at all stages of life is wise beyond words! It can't be overstated. When Claire took food discipline seriously, her weight flew off and the figure she had at goal was exceptional. It wasn't just a number that pleased her. Exercise does that.

TRAPS: Losing weight for someone else is not a promising premise. Luckily, Claire shifted to her own desire to do this. But, often it doesn't play out that way. It's usually a sign there's some deeper problem in the relationship. Lose for you.

CHARLOTTE:

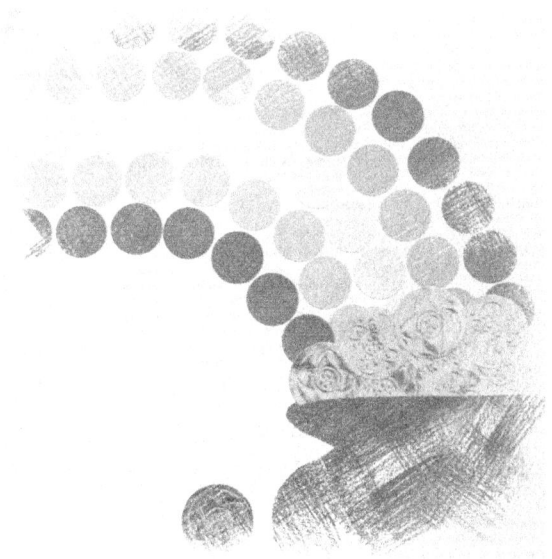

Charlotte joined the program at a very low point in her life. Her family had lost their home to foreclosure in the downturned economy. Moving from place to place with 2 teenagers combined with her husband's employment being unstable was a combination for stress and uncertainty.

Far more serious: her own health. Charlotte had battled internal surgeries that would take a toll on anyone. Let alone someone who's life was in turmoil, already. Emotionally, it took a very strong woman to bear the daily strain. Physically, she had to relearn how to eat. Many restrictions kept eating a daily challenge to discover, sometimes painfully, what digested comfortably and what was off limits. Many would have seen the extra weight as either unfixable or just ignored it because her life was so hard, in general. Not Charlotte.

She joined the program determined to not use any of these disadvantages as an excuse. I admire her spirit. Trial and error would be the way she'd navigated her new life and it would be the road map here, too. Weekly, she'd be in class contributing, listening, make adjustments as needed and the weight came off. The occasional gain was taken in its stride. Her sensible and patient outlook saw her through all these potential roadblocks. She even began to see her inability to eat certain things as a blessing. I knew we could work together since we were both willing to be so flexible.

A new job came Charlotte's way. She looks fantastic. Her kids are becoming fine young adults and her husband remained a supportive element. This lady's transformation against seriously difficult circumstances only makes the slim, beautiful person she now is more of a joy to witness. I am confident she will remain the 'new her' forevermore.

TIPS: If you think personal setbacks make weight loss impossible, Charlotte slayed that excuse, didn't she? She was willing to put more time, research and effort into this as necessary byproducts of her circumstances and tackled it.

TRAPS: Charlotte didn't fall into any! I can only mirror what she did NOT do - use her health as a barrier. Will your road be harder, slow, and have more pitfalls? Perhaps, it must. But can you still decide to lose weight and better yourself –yes!

OLIVIA:

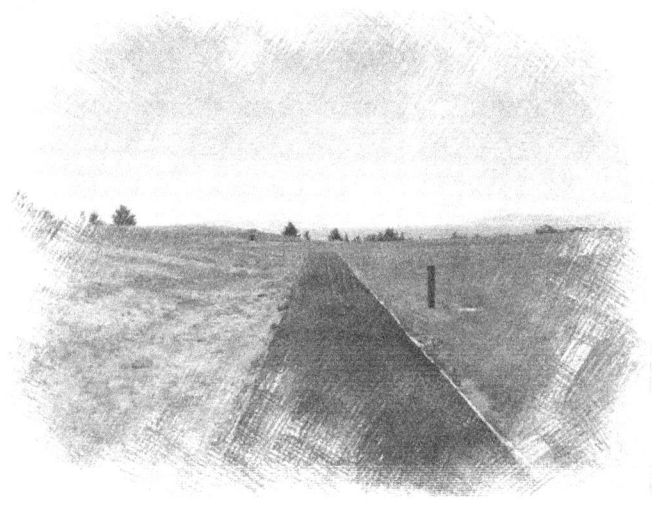

I have had every region of the world blamed for why someone was overweight. You don't understand, I'm Polish - we eat! We're Italian - we eat! We're Latin - we eat! We're Swedish - we eat! We're Jewish - we eat! We're Tongan - we eat! You get the picture. On the national landscape: I'm Southern - we eat! I'm from the Midwest - we eat! I'm from New Orleans, Chicago, New York, San Francisco, Memphis - we eat! OK, let me add mine: I'm Greek - we eat, too. As opposed to where? Tell me where do people not eat? Those lucky stiffs in Canada, Indonesia, Uruguay and the Maldives Islands - they live on oxygen, right? You'll never challenge yourself to get thin if you set up permanent camp there. That excuse is designed to ensure you make no progress. You can't change your nationality or upbringing. I could have remained obese forever with that one. So can you.

This is how I met Olivia. Let's throw a dart at the map and hear another one: Olivia was from the South - they eat! Fried is so common there that grilled or baked or broiled foods were about as familiar to Olivia as colors are to a person born blind. It's hard to explain this objectively. I am lucky. While I was given many fattening foods and developed my own tastes for more and devious ways to get them, I also like healthy food. So, abandoning the junk didn't leave me as stranded as it does some people. No one likes feeling stranded. Olivia was one of those people. At least 100# overweight at 26 years old, she dressed like an older person, spoke very quietly, walked slowly and was taking medication for health troubles that she was far too young for. I'll never forget her comment that the only fresh veggies she'd likely ever had were on top of hamburgers or pizza. Wow. At least she was being honest.

Another problem for Olivia was that she did have a particular health malady. This made some meds necessary but was also a crutch Olivia used to give up and not try where she could make improvements. Her passive nature was her biggest obstacle. She identified with how overweight I'd been and began to strike a pleasant weekly rapport with me that I enjoyed, too. Often members that are quite overweight find they prefer a teacher who's been in their shoes. They don't feel a person who took off 30 or less pounds, while admirable, is going to help them through some challenges because they simply cannot know the massive difference there is in being as obese as they are. I understand this. My teacher had taken off 60+#. I don't think I would have bonded with a 25 or less pounds lost person, either. Olivia began opening up to me and I found her youth there. She was in her 20s and spoke like a typical young girl with more 'likes' in between her sentences than this English Lit major cares to hear. She liked hip hop music and country line dancing and although she was unable to do it, I told her to use that as a light to strive towards. She beamed with hope!

Still, the struggle between the angel on one shoulder and the demon on the other was a rough one for Olivia. Her losses were not what they could be because she was hit and miss with her habits. Junk food, sweets and baking were all so engrained in her and the withdrawal too much for her and she'd cave often. I never tisk-tisked her for that, it's not productive and not my style. But I had to give her the feedback that she simply couldn't expect change with no long term effort on her part and that a 50/50 approach wasn't gonna work. She didn't disagree because I know she knew that was right, but she wasn't willing to put the action into this. On and on her weight never got too far.

I found out Olivia was on full disability and earned babysitting money. A woman in her 20s on full disability because working caused her anxiety and stress and her health was used as a caveat by her physician and there she was, apparently set up for a government supported existence for the next 50 years. My respect for her dropped. I am human and am allowed my own private thoughts. I never shared this with Olivia, but a part of my concern for her diminished the night I discovered that. Olivia was lazy. I couldn't tap dance around it anymore. This required work and she was lazy. No reward for that. Babysitting for extra spending money at 27 while collecting a check under dubious circumstances, please!

Now, that doesn't mean I didn't still like Olivia and was fully willing to help her. But my patience with her excuses was near gone. One night with a disappointing weigh in, Olivia looked very glum and I approached her and she asked if we could talk after the meeting some. She said sure. I wear many hats in my class - therapist, pastor in the confessional, open ear friend being a few of them. I still cared about Olivia, no matter how little she was doing on her own behalf.

She spoke of her frustration on not losing weight. This was expected. I gave her the same style talk we'd had before about how her blaming her Southern upbringing had to end, her attempts at keeping fattening foods that are too tempting in her house were not a wise idea, her fast food addiction had to be put on hold and she gave the usual   look-at-the-floor-because-I-don't-like-what-he's-saying-but-I-know-it's-true-so-I-kinda-have-to-not-argue I've seen in many members. I gave it to many teachers in my day.

She told me that she'd gone out with friends to see a rap concert the past weekend. I asked if it was a good show and she said the best part was when the hunky rapper took his shirt off. I laughed. I saw a potential opening here to help Olivia. She'd said many times how her single status was bothersome when all her girlfriends were married or attached. Of course, this was because of how heavy she was and men were so stupid and shallow and didn't see the good soul and heart in a woman like her. Poor me scenarios are not good for motivation. I pointed out to her that she liked the hunky rapper most when he took his shirt off. SHE wasn't attracted to heavy men, was she? "Eww, NO!' she replied. HA! She was just as shallow as anyone. Did she have any desire to look deeper into the soul of the double chinned men she saw? No. This seemed to hit like a magic bullet, avoiding all her defenses and excuses and hitting Olivia right in the heart. A revelation: she was too young to be this heavy and nothing was going to get better as she aged unless she attacked this problem. She got a fire in her that I'd never seen before.

A few months of weight loss and, while not perfect, a better track record and willing mind to change were Olivia's motto. I was hopeful, too. Then, one day she had to tell me she couldn't come to classes anymore for financial reasons. This I cannot dig too deeply into unless it's offered by the members since it's not my business. I wanted to say, "You seemed to have money for candy, McDonalds, cinnamon rolls, booze and concert tickets, but not this?" I stilled my tongue. Olivia wasn't ready. Maybe the money thing was true - it didn't matter. If she'd won a lottery, Olivia wasn't ready. I wasn't ready in my 20s and went through many unhappy, unhealthy years, icky experiences and no experiences you should have in other areas before I would be. With all my heart I hope Olivia chooses to save herself.

TIPS: If Olivia did one thing right, it was reaching out to me. She didn't sit and stew over her problems. Also, she came and told me to my face when she was quitting. That was a very admirable thing. Very few do this. We KNOW how to quit - you weasel away and don't look back.

TRAPS: Lazy won't do. It just isn't designed to. Examine yourself and decide if you're willing to work very hard, mentally and physically. No one can do this on lazy mode.

GUY AND NORA:

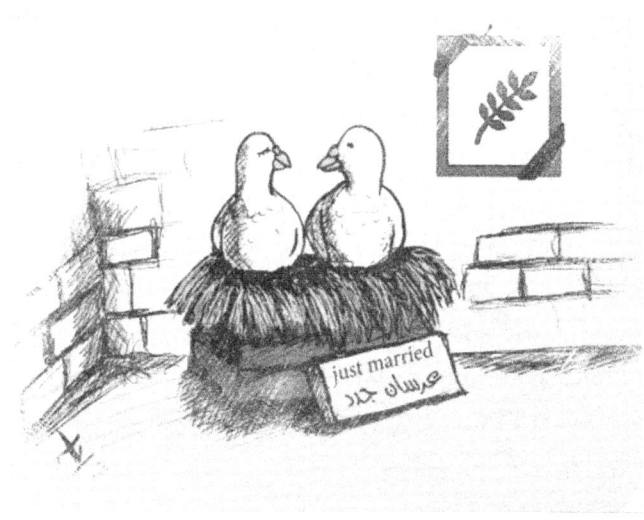

One of the opportunities the program offers is meetings brought to your place of business. The convenience of having on sight classes is its main selling point. It was in one of those off center locales that I met Guy and Nora, a couple from the Midwest who were both 100# overweight. They were both quite congenial and seemed eager to take off their considerable excess poundage by being compliant to the program - another case of my easiest type of new members. Welcome!

They began with the kind of story I am familiar with. The upbringing of one's life sets the tone for how food is emphasized, prepared and dictates flavor preferences, too. Just as I've had nationality blamed for poor eating habits and naturally big boned people, I've heard regions of the United States made the scapegoat. The South certainly takes top prize for this, but the Midwest has its shame-ers, too.

There's good reason it's referred to as America's bread basket - those folks like bread. They eat lots of it. Midwestern people often generationally pass this habit on and Guy and Nora were no exceptions. Both spoke of the gravies, biscuits, corn on the cob, butter drenched meat loaf comfort foods they gorged on all their lives: starch bloat 101. It seems the reality check of 'you can't eat like farmers did in past decades when you're not doing the physical labor they were doing' doesn't always occur to them, it needs spelled out sometimes. When I pinpoint this honest truth out, I ask - "Do you work in your farm as hard as your parents did?" No. "Did you work as hard on your farm as your grandparents did?" Not even close. "Then you can't EAT like they did."

The job transfer that had taken them out West gave them the chance to view other types of eating and cuisine and to modify their ways, but they didn't change. They ate like they'd gotten off the farm last week instead of 30 years ago. You have to work at staying that insulated. These were not sheltered people. They were both very intelligent, too. They were, however, unimaginative people who had ignored their bodies too long, but at least freely admitted it. I could work with them.

The main difference between Guy and Nora was that Guy acclimated to Las Vegas. Nora resisted it. "I'll never say I'm from here. I'm a little girl from the Midwest and I'll say that 'til the day I die even if we live here for the next 30 years." There had to be a willingness to dive into the program forward focused or the odds would not be with them. They gave me their word they would and I believed them. That is a trait I love about Midwestern people that I've known. They tell it like it is. There aren't layers of drama to them usually. That works in their favor. Guy and Nora both began losing weight quickly and worked well together. Truly, a husband and wife team on the same page. No jealousy or competition or sneaking behind one's back with them. As they lost weight and began seeing numbers they'd not seen in most of their married life, it was like seeing 60-year-old kids getting their most wished for present on their birthdays. I looked forward to seeing them weekly. They very rarely missed.

Particularly to Nora's advantage was her fondness for cooking was adaptable. She bought many cookbooks but unlike too many members, she used them. Nora just didn't know how to cook basic tasty nutritious food. That's a very teachable skill. Seasonings proved her new toys. Raised on butter, salt, mayonnaise, Crisco oil, ketchup and not much else - I saw her open her pallet to spices I was versatile with and made entrees, breakfasts, salads, variations on her standard comfort foods and baked goods. They came alive because of her thoroughness and tenacity. People have often given up on themselves when I meet them, Nora was discovering her ability to change fundamental habits and it gave her a big confidence boot! Healthy food could taste good - WOW! Guy joked he'd never had meals with explanations for what was in them in their entire marriage. He was a co- operative man that wanted to make the changes easy for the two of them and happily ate the dishes his wife prepared and shared in her later in life realizations about new flavors.

Well, armed with this and the program, pounds came off very steadily. Guy ended up 100+#s lighter and Nora, as well. What a pair!

Shopping was a joy to Nora and an annoyance for Guy - ironically for the same reason. Nora loved having choices that plus size stores didn't allow. Jeans, coats, button blouses, clam diggers - whatever Nora wanted and in sizes that didn't depress her made her glow with pride. Guy didn't like shopping and found the rut of only buying the one thing or so that fit him in the big men's stores convenient. HA! What a problem to have! The choices available meant time spent in department stores looking around, trying on things, making decisions based on more than what fits were all drudgery for him. No worries. His wife loved shopping for him, too. Really he trusted her taste - he was most amazed at the sizes when she'd tell him he was in size 38 slacks, or a size large sweater or even smaller size shoes. Yes, many people have that drop, too. When there's less weight pressing down on them, many members' feet retake their natural form and suddenly, their shoes don't fit. I went from an 11 wide to a 10 1/2 regular. I'm glad I didn't know I had foot fat. I was self-conscious enough.

At goal for Guy, he tried to downplay the attention on him (modesty is another common Midwestern attribute). He said, "I don't give a damn how I look. Never have." While I was trying to find the words to build him up and let him let himself see what a big deal he'd done - Nora started crying. Why, I asked. "His face, I haven't seen that face in over 35 years. He looks like the man I married. Except for gray hair, this is the groom I saw as I walked down the aisle. While it's always been in my heart, it's as though a time machine has put that face back on my husband and I'm seeing my young groom again." Well, there wasn't a dry eye in the room and Guy turned away so his own welled up tears could be unseen. What a great reward. Guy was speechless as he walked over to his loving wife, embraced her and said he'd never seen a change in all their years together. She was eternally the young bride he'd married in his eyes no matter what her age, weight or anything else.

Now, what food tastes good enough to deny yourself a moment like that? No food in the world. Even the readers who just mentioned a food under your breath - yea, I know you did - you're wrong. I say that because you can eat any food you like - in moderation and still have an outcome like Guy and Nora. What are you waiting for?

TIPS: Teamwork! They are candidates for the best example of it I've seen. Being willing to be reeducated in cooking was indispensable for Nora, too. It's only food. It only takes an open mind to learn.

TRAPS: Passivity. It kept Guy and Nora heavy much longer than it needed to. You must not oblige any acceptance of your state - or it won't change.

KELLY:

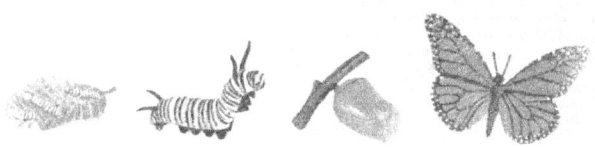

How can I begin about Kelly? She's awesome. That's a good beginning. She's thin and happy. That's a good end. Now, for the in-between: she came to me already 70+ pounds lighter. The class she's been attending was cancelled and only out of necessity did we meet. Blond, fair skinned and wholesome looking, her achievement was already quite admirable.

But I found that she and I could connect for the remainder of her weight loss journey. You see, Kelly still had a good 60 more pounds to lose. She'd been considerably overweight. Her before picture was unrecognizable. She was very fond of her previous teacher. I knew that woman and we're very different in personality and style. She'd moved out of town and wasn't coming back. My work would be cut out for me to win her trust and accept a coach change mid game.

She was very shy and didn't want attention paid to her accomplishments. Man, being overweight is a confidence killer. She should have been tooting her own horn loudly and proudly. Instead, she sat unsmiling, wearing Granny sweaters FAR too early in life. But, she was listening. I could see that. I know when I'm being listened to and when I'm being semi listened to and when I'm being dismissed. Our bond began to get strong because I also had lost weight in the numbers she was facing. I gave her extra time privately before or after meetings. She shared her struggles with adjusting to the attention her weight loss was naturally drawing. You can't lose the amount she had and expect people to not notice. She was uncomfortable with attention, particularly positive attention. I understood. I admired her tenacity.

I also took a bit of a risk in leveling with her that while her weight drop was big, she wasn't thin. Nowhere near it. MANY people fall into a premature sense of complacency when they've lost a lot of weight. It's an easy trap to fall in. You look better, you feel better, people are complimenting you, you're in clothing sizes you either haven't been in your entire life or in a number of years .... BUT you're not thin. It's not time to do the victory dance on the 20-yard line. There's a place you need a good objective teacher to keep you going forward. Too, too many drop off this way. My perspective by meeting her 2/3 of the way through the journey helped with this. Although I could see a picture and know how great she'd done. My first impression of her was not with this information. I saw a woman who was 50# overweight. She wanted to be thin - all the way. I became her co-pilot.

Kelly followed me through 3 location changes. What a trooper! She'd connected with me and that was it! I always objectively tell members that they're free agents to go to any location, day, time or try on new teachers. No one can be the right fit for everyone. But, I must say I was glad and very humbly flattered at her, 'No way, it's your classes

I'm going to, I don't care where you are, I'm staying with you!' stance. With each class and location change she became more relaxed and opened up to the class more. She made new friends. It was so nice to see. Her numbers went past 100#, 105, 110 and the class began to recognize her as the harbinger of wisdom every time she spoke, which was every class.

She always kept honest and real. No one loses this weight and has a perfect life. Overweight people can sometimes idealize being thin as an end all / be all nirvana. I know I certainly used to see it that way when I was on the 'outside looking in'. I know differently now. Kelly had trouble with her friends. They were unsupportive of her success and quite jealous. They tried to criticize her and told her she was getting too thin and that she looked sick ... what nerve! I cannot tell you how often I hear examples of this. I often say, 'You want to find out who your friends are? Lose a lot of weight. See who's supportive and see who gets weird.' Most members have people land on both sides of this scenario. I did. Kelly, too. It saddened me. It's their own inability to do the work that they're turning outward in a nasty way at the person who's changing their life.

Kelly took off more than 150#! The class gave her a standing ovation. I made her promise she'd keep attending. Like the honest person she is, she said she would and is in class every week working on the tough road of maintaining. I have seen her wear bright colors, younger styles, jeans (!), make up, cool shoes and shine with an inner self satisfaction that becomes her. I hear her friends never came around and still try to put her down. Why she remains friends with them, I don't know. It's not my business.

Kelly is a shining example of the best the program can offer some-one. Her life is literally transformed. She continues the work and I have no doubt this is the lady shall be from now on!

TIPS: It's not productive to put a teacher before the les-sons needed to be learned. In Kelly's case, it proved nec-essary for her to accept a coach change and two location changes. Change isn't easy for some. Thankfully, Kelly isn't one to be stopped.

TRAPS: It hurts my heart when friends prove unworthy of us. It's a big disappointment and most cannot keep con-nected to the person. Kelly continues seeing hers and takes arrows regularly. I'd have cut them out of my life, but I'm not Kelly. I feel so badly for her. LET GO of unsupportive peo-ple. Alone is better than toxic company.

LARRY:

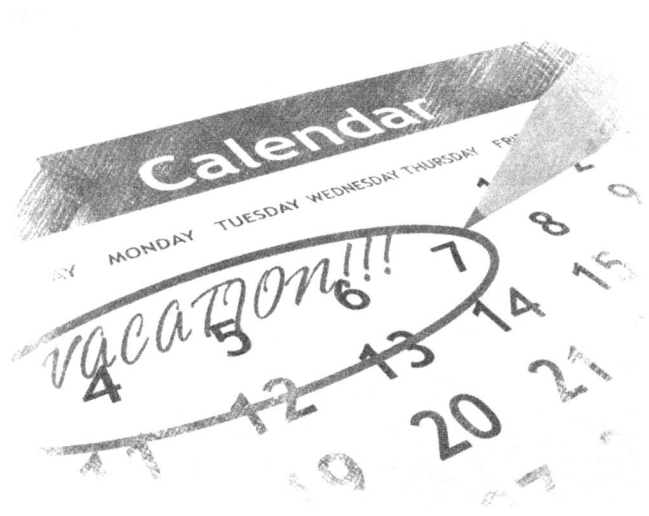

Some folks take good advice and avoid trouble. Other people have to test it and learn the hard way. The school of hard knocks isn't an easy one to endure. But, I've enrolled unwillingly in it before. I suppose most of us do, from time to time. As a teacher, I spew a lot of advice. I always make sure I back up anything I say with fact: facts from reliable sources, reputable nutritional news, up to the minute advances in science and, most of all, personal life experience - always the best teacher. No one needs to pay good money to sit and hear anyone's two cents. I respect my members enough to share the truths.

Not everyone appreciates hearing the truth. Some members shop teachers until they find one that says what they want to hear. I do not connect well with those types. It's not in my nature to play my part in that game and so I must risk ruffling feathers sometimes. Most often, they know it is accurate information.

A good example: needing to keep program on vacations. That does not always go over well. Vacations are supposed to be free for all's with food and drink. Eat and drink yourself into oblivion is how they intend to spend their vacations and I'm a wet blanket on their fun. Well, no wonder they're ticked when I try to play the rational level headed tune they don't want to hear. Cruises had claimed many people's progress as they lay in the sun enjoying the endless offers of abundant food and libation. Without food, they can't relax or enjoy. After all, isn't that what vacations are for?

It's a habit: a deeply ingrained habit for some. I, too, have enjoyed several holidays where every meal was a festival of overeating. I have returned with 10 pounds on in one week and pants that fit on Sunday that were barely buttonable on Saturday. Never bothered me, either, it was normal and expected. The program challenges us to rethink normal and what is expected on a daily basis. This is an area some members find very tough to rewrite.

I connect our principles often with what's taught in 12 step meetings and this is a key to trying to persuade members to keep vacations sensible. When you're an alcoholic, you don't get pre permission to fall off the wagon on vacations. Gamblers cannot return to casinos. Drug addicts cannot get high.... but, gluttony is another matter. It's not restricted and everyone has to eat and it's great for business. So, the tourist eating their way through road trips is a win/win for many people. If only it were that easy.

The trouble is when you return home, you cannot shut it off like a light bulb. If that were possible, then you don't have to join the program and I wish you well. I'm here for the afflicted that find it impossible to walk the middle area. Cross addiction is common and the logic transfers well from one substance to another. When I ask classes if they're tried that rationale that they'll 'just let go' while they're on vacation and get right back on their diets when they return, many hands go up. When I follow up with, 'and who did that NOT work out for?', every hand stays up.

It was a relearning of what to do with yourself on vacations from square one for me. It was humbling to see how food focused my life was that I had not a clue what to do for a whole week if food wasn't the top priority. A deflating sense of 'Why bother going?' choked at my resolve. Only my determination to keep going forward with this or never take a vacation again got me to delve into other strategies to have fun without overeating. This is a common lesson for addicts in recovery. I can and do make plans that are fun, cultural, relaxing or whatever my vacation destination takes me. But, it was learned behavior.

To be honest, I cannot un-know the joy of unchecked eating being the main purpose of vacations past and the fun they can be. But, like the drinker that must face the hangover, the gambler that must face his bills, the addict that must come down off their high, I had to reignite my fire by remembering the damage. That helps me a great deal. Members seem to gravitate to this.

Well, SOME do. I know I'm preaching to deaf ears to some of them. They leave going 'that was a lot of nonsense. If he thinks I'm gonna go to and not eat, he's crazy.' As if I were a fly on the wall, I know.

That's why I need members to share their stories. I know that the same points can be made by the 'teacher' and it'll be discounted by many because 'the teacher said it'. When a fellow member says it, suddenly it's got some merit. This may disappoint the teacher in me, but the realist says wherever the true information comes from, if it's accepted and applied, it's alright.

Larry was a big man with a big voice and personality. He was hit and miss with weight loss but his heart was in the right place. He really did want to do the right thing, but the pull of the food was just so strong and his will didn't always succeed. But, he never made excuses and seemed willing to get back up and try again. I love that trait in members. Larry was a great guy. With about 50% of his weight off, he'd gone on a vacation. In the season that passed, it was not going well for Larry. He got quieter and sat in the back more often. A busy meeting, I didn't push him to talk since I know that often back-fires. One fateful night, Larry raised his hand when the subject of vacationing on program was being suggested by me and resisted by most. He said, I was doing well on the program and lost 60#. Feeling great, I decided I would take the week off for a vacation. I deserved it. It was a vacation. I'd get right back on after that. Well, it's been 5 months and it was the biggest mistake of my life." Larry's voice began to rise and crack. 'I have never been able to fully get my mojo back. Try as I may, it has never been the same. That one week off program is long gone and I'm still suffering for it. I regret it so much. If I had it to do over again, I'd have listened to you, ALL of you - don't do it. My faith in myself is shaky and I think about quitting all the time now. ALL for one week off." The room was silent. I quietly said that it took courage, Larry sized courage to open up to the room like that and that we needed to adhere his good advice and thank him for sharing. ALL of you owe him a debt if your next vacation goes well, now. The room applauded. Larry never did recapture his fire.

You take your DNA with you! It doesn't play that game with us. "Oh, you're in another time zone? I see, well, I'll just not absorb calories or fat until you get back home." Don't we wish? If learning how to live life with food not being #1 means re-examining everything, that's where you'll need to start. One week that's compromised is bearable because the other 51 in a year are great. That's how I cope. I have many new memories that'll last a lifetime that would never have been done because they were too vigorous or too inconvenient or too out of the way or too bathing suit oriented before. Food, you didn't defeat me. That's an all year vacation. Larry, I hope you found your fire, again.

TIPS: Short term sacrifice for long term payoffs is de rigueur for weight loss. Vacations often are testing grounds for this. Look up where you're going and see what non-food oriented things there are to do there. I promise you - there are.

TRAPS: Re-writing your primary living guides is a daunting task. Many just won't do it. Vacations will always trip you up if you're unprepared. Regret will follow you all next season.

VICKI:

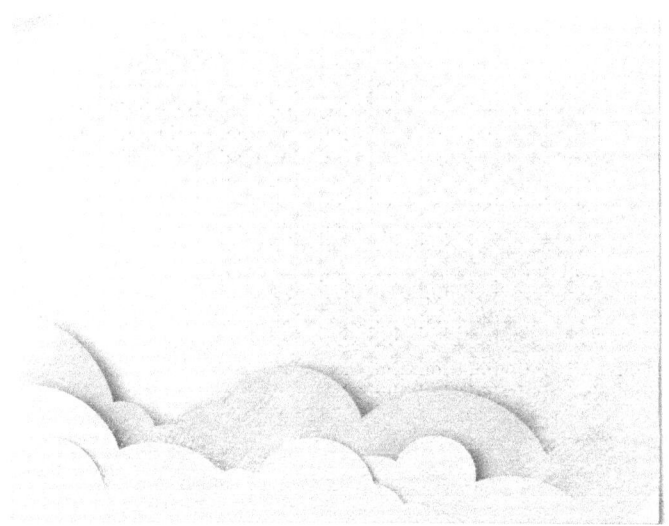

Vicki was a pleasant type. I like pleasant types. I'm so unimpressed with cynicism. Negative people who only look at the bleak side, that never seem to be having a good day, take perverse delight in things not working out for others, vent their anger at those around them trying to better themselves...just 'glass is half empty, at best' folks. Usually, it's challenging to be in their company. I am related to a few. I avoid them.

Vicki again reinforced my high opinion of women, seniors and people trying this against situations not of their own causing. Vicki was in all of these categories. Vicki was short, so the extra 30# was enough to impact her life in ways she was just sick and tired of enough to do something about it. THAT'S when I can work with someone best. That's the easiest two team lift off point I can ask for.

Vicki made my job easier by joining the program pre agreed that she couldn't do it alone, she needed to adopt a permanent lifestyle change and that she'd attend classes and follow up. Wow, I wanted to clone her. You never know what's going on in a person's life by the 'mask' we all put on for the public. As I said, Vicki was a relaxed and happy lady who complained very rarely and had that 'roll up your sleeves, pitch in when there's work to be done and keep griping to a minimum' that's not as prevalent in younger generations. Our Loss: it's an incredibly useful way to navigate life.

Vicki liked the accountability of the weekly weigh in and having me look at her journal. Each member must decide how they're going to react to the needed steps to thin. You can make this as easy or hard as possible. The weekly weigh in is essential. It is absolutely essential. You behave differently. It's proven to me over and over again. Members returning or first timers alike need it. People who get thin too often make the huge mistake of retreating from it the moment they're at goal. The need to embrace it is vital for anyone. As for the journals being shown to me, I don't force it. If a member wants extra accountability I'm glad to oblige. I give myself much extra work by offering to take any members' journals and go over them to find suggestions, question entries that seem inaccurate or challenge notions that they're simply not losing weight but doing the program right. It's my sincere desire to see everyone succeed at this. The overtime comes with the caring.

It was with no judging that Vicki gave her trackers to me. In fact, she thrived on it. Knowing I'd be there expecting it made her better. Slimmer and slimmer Vicki went from the back row at class #1 to the front row by the time goal was imminent. I've watched with glee as this locale change manifested inner growth often. I usually don't jinx it by saying a word. Sometimes, just letting the good habits evolve in their natural progression is the most supportive thing a teacher can do. Vicki beamed with pride.

Vicki also took this later in life confidence to the karate dojo! Many members take up new hobbies they either always wanted to do or discovered they wanted with dewy new confidence. Never one to let her age, gender, size or any other obstacle deter her, Vicki took up martial arts at over 60 and earned a black belt. This was reacted to in a room FULL of women 55 and over with amazement. She was taking the excuses out and replacing them with her new life. This was a role model for all of them. I know some of them were inspired to do their parts more proactively under Vicki's shining example. She drove all over the Southwest to tournaments to compete. When you're in a fringe sport or category, you cannot have the action come to you. You often have to go to it. There is not an abundance of women over 60 fighting in karate tournaments. So, only the diehard practitioners are usually there. I pity the purse snatcher that tries to mess with her. You rock, Vicki.

Vicki made goal and with ease like a superstar. Like the good student she is, Vicki kept attending classes, getting weighed and working to keep her weight down. As I'd said, you don't know what's going on in someone's world unless they invite you in. Vicki made it look easy. Looks can be deceiving. The only glimpse of trouble she'd shared was that her husband was not overweight and didn't intend to alter his eating and that meant she had to create 2 meals 3 times a day that included tempting foods for her. Another case of men getting away with this because the woman in their life complies: ridiculous! Well, I suppose, as an outsider, I am not of a useful opinion. I'm told those types of compromise are necessary if you want to stay married. That's why I'm single, I guess. Vicki was more of a warrior than I'd already thought.

Her family is all overweight. Her daughter struggled with her weight, came in and out of the program without success and made her mother feel very awkward over doing so much better than her, too. I truly don't like people who see others shine and instead of trying to rise to their level, throw mud at them to bring them down so that they don't feel badly about their own lack of discipline. Awful behavior! Families! Vicki had never let on that she was battling this civil unrest all during her loss. I don't know how she did it. I don't know if I could have. I take that back. I know I couldn't have.

After years of smooth maintaining weight, Vicki began to struggle. Now, visibly shaken, she opened up that her husband was struggling with some terminal disease and that she was taking care of him 24/7 and that her weight was up and that she was close to throwing in the towel. She did love this man very much. His diagnosis was not my business unless she offered. I didn't probe. I knew my part in this lay with Vicki. He didn't help her in the best of circumstances. I was sure he wouldn't help her now. I offered an open ear, a willingness to let her talk about what was scaring her and only suggested weight loss tactics if she wanted them.

The good sense Vicki has served her well again. She got back to goal again and will never allow personal tragedies to take her away from her own health and sanity again. I was proud of her from the beginning. When she told me of her struggles that she'd had during that time, I was prouder of her. Recapturing goal by returning to her teacher and admitting she'd slipped up and taking the weight back off again - wow. Vicki, I respectfully bow to you.

TIPS: Enrich your life in ways you've only dreamed of. This is how your transition to a thin-for-life person unfolds. In some cases, it's something you never knew you wanted or would be good at. Put in the order - One new life, TO GO!

TRAPS: Accommodating unsupportive people helps no one. They don't change because they don't have to. Vicki has the strength of a super hero. I don't. Unless you think you do, this will be a landmine waiting to blow up constantly. When my mother quit smoking, she told my father he had to smoke outdoors. He should have also quit smoking, but that's a personal decision you cannot make someone do. But, she told him he wasn't going to puff in her face. Knowing objecting to a determined Mediterranean woman is absolutely futile; he smoked outside for the rest of his life.

ASHLEY:

REPEAT AFTER ME:
"I CAN DO THIS"

Ashley was a likeable lady from the moment we met. She joined with her husband and we hit it off immediately. It was mutual like. Both of them were in their 30s and overweight enough to be a concern that was to be addressed as a team. Both of Latin decent, they had personality and a wide range of interests, particularly, Ashley. Working in public relations, catering, party-planning as careers suited her perfectly. Her enthusiasm was the kind you cannot teach. She had a contagious happy vibe that would enhance anyone's functions or party. She dressed with sass and flair - a trait I love and wanted to do the program so she could shed the weight that was bringing her down.

Her husband was less gregarious, but very friendly, too. It would have been next to impossible to be more outgoing, so I suppose happy cool was his best role. The two of them were an ideal situation as far as couples go. Most of the time, one does much better than the other and it causes friction. This is true with most twosomes no matter what their relation. I only told them the basics at their orientation: such as men lose faster than women, she had to account for her time of the month, he was taller. .... Ashley knew all this and didn't seem worried. She didn't even make any of the standard replies about how much luckier men are with any resentment in her tone. Negativity wasn't in her vocabulary - Let's DO this!

They were an education for me, as well. I have known many Latin people. I'd hear that the women are naturally curvy and that Caucasian measurements were unrealistic to aspire to. Ashley was curvy, indeed. It was her born build. What she wasn't going to let happen was it being an excuse to not be as thin as she could. She told me of how many of her fellow Latina friends accepted a weight higher than they should be. I wanted to take a higher degree of interest in Ashley to help her prove this right.

Exercise wasn't an obstacle - Zumba classes and Salsa dancing were fun for her. She would benefit from this and as the extra weight came off, there was already muscle ready to be shown off. There was no need for Ashley to come out of a shell - she was in no shell. Her make-up, jewelry, hair, shoes were all well thought out and stylish. She needed motivation and some basic education the program could provide. She and her husband took joy in rearranging traditional Spanish cuisine into lower calorie, fat and carb recipes that were still tasty and kept their authenticity. I listened with great interest as I found out healthier ways to enjoy carne Asada, Chile con carne, flautas and other things too many people forego when they go on diets. These 2 were not on a diet.

Ashley's husband made goal first, Ashley soon after: what a team!! They were each other's biggest fan and never showed the slightest bit of jealousy or competition. This is why they had their winning outcomes. I knew they'd be a smooth ride for them. When I was told Ashley was pregnant, I knew I was only saying 'So Long' until she gave birth. Pregnant women are not allowed in the program. Her husband continued to attend and kept me posted on her progress. 9 months later, a baby boy was added to their family.

Ashley came back. Let's DO this, again. While never less than the upbeat delight she'd always been, Ashley struggled this time. Not one to make excuses, she never blamed having recently had a baby for it. It was just the same simple struggle we all have - food tastes good and we love eating it. That's why any of us join the program. Temptations were hard to resist. Her own life could throw her curves, but she was going to persevere. This was going to be tested more than she may have known.

Ashley and her husband went through difficult financial times and had to downsize, such a pity. It was the common story in Nevada for far too many people. I was sad to hear this happen to good folks like them. Job changes: Ashley went through some career changes from a big company to a smaller one and this is often challenging. To my surprise, she and her husband divorced. You never know what's going on in someone's private life. I was sorry to hear this. I cannot say that I'd ever disliked him, but I only saw the surface. I believe Ashley is a sincere person and made necessary, but difficult choices. Most challenging of all, her son was a special needs child. What a load to bear: if you believe God doesn't give anyone more than they can handle: Ashley can handle tremendous amounts of trials at once.

Now, this combination does one of two things to a person. You can become an angry, cynical, ball of negativity that shouts bile to anyone who gets near you. It can make you hate the opposite gender forever, shake your faith to its core and defeat your will. This trek predictably takes one down a road to a bitter person that may cope by overeating and gives up any hope of being thin forever. Ashley didn't do this. She chose the opposite.

A classy lady to the core: she never overshared her woes in the meeting, bashed her ex-husband or made too much of her career taking new directions that would involve trying times when you see what fits. Her son was the light of her life and the prime focus of her existence. She was determined to be the Ashley she was beforehand: A fun, cool, kind, stylish, proud young woman who embraced life and drew good people to her. She rolled up her sleeves and makes the best life for her son she can. Social media kept us all abreast of his progress and her ability to be as proud of his achievements as all parents are. While her son will take extra care and effort as he grows, I know he'll get all he needs to be a strong, confident and happy with a warrior mother like Ashley.

While there's a road full of more trials than most parents will go through ahead for Ashley, I know as surely as I type this that she's up for it. She'll get thin, she' raise a fine man, she'll salsa dance and inspire anyone whom she invites to her party.

TIPS: Relearn foods you grew up with. It's not impossible. Just learn tweaks to old comfort foods and, POW, you're eating them again. Ashley expects support. No boyfriend will be tolerated if he doesn't.

TRAPS: Ashley didn't fall into any. I've rarely seen anyone have so many tough blows thrown at them and remain strong, successful and smiling as her.

ZELDA:

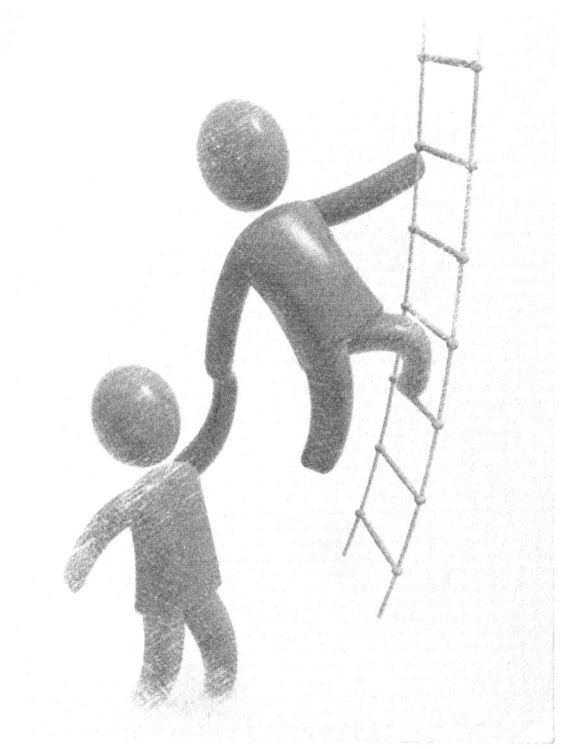

Zelda, my teacher, what a woman! What a broad is a better description. Don't get me wrong, those of you who are fluent in politically correct speaking. You've probably already realized I alternate between PC and non PC as the story dictates. I mean 'broad' in the best way! Brassy, confident, appreciated a good time, dressed to show off her best assets, unapologetic to those who may not agree with her or tested her patience too long.

I found Zelda looking for a new teacher. I joined looking to change my life and with the right attitude and all that. However, I cannot over emphasize how crucial the right connection with the right teacher is. Since the program is still the program no matter who teaches it, some may say it doesn't matter. I do respectfully disagree. How the class is conducted and the information passed plays a great part in most people continuing the journey all the way to goal.

Case in point, I wasn't crazy for my first teacher. She was very popular, so I was obviously not in the majority opinion. Reasons: she wasn't really thin! I want a teacher who is at goal and is walking the walk. Not just talking the talk. Reasons: her whole 'schpiel', if you will, wasn't my style, a cowgirl who adopted a Minnie Pearl kind of hokey 'Howdy, y'all' delivery that this West coast man couldn't relate to or find amusing or engaging. Reasons: her manners were not up to snuff! She inhaled her mucus when she talked. She was a blunt talker and that trait I take just fine. But only if there's help with your dilemmas. She wasn't so good with follow up help. Reasons: she went on and on about her daughter, friends .... while I like personal sharing it's only beneficial if it tweaks the class to be involved or has points of learning behind the story. There were never any. She just rambled (often, through entire classes). Final straw reason: low key celebrating. I like to toot my horn and those of others. She often woefully underplayed weight losses or forgot to even get to them due to her fascinating stories. When you hit 25#, a magnet is issued. I was so proud of myself. She'd neglected to ask anyone about milestone accomplishments during the meeting. So, afterwards, I went up to her to ask for the magnet and I mentioned that she'd not made time for celebrations. She replied a sarcastic toned, "So, you need a piece of plastic to feel like you lost weight?" or something close to that effect. The precise words are possibly wrong, but the message is spot on. That was it. The heck with her and her corn pone act.

I knew I'd like Zelda when I walked in the door with her high, copper hair on a made up face of a smiling businesswoman. Her tailored suit was accessorized attractively and the black pencil skirt showed off some seriously good looking legs. A pair of high heels combined to make her over six feet tall. She put effort into this look. She was dressed to go to a cocktail party or a night club at 4:30 in the afternoon. Whew, I'm ready to get to goal with this one.

Zelda was also a blunt talker, but gave constructive advice and guidance. For these who told her that their half-hearted efforts were not paying off-- they'd be treated to a 'why are you surprised? You've mentioned this before. It didn't work last month and it won't work next month, either.' Ha! Right! She inspired me to be better, be prepared, take notes, to follow up on assignments she'd suggest. I sat in the front and spoke often. I also listened. I never left one class feeling like it was a waste of time or money.

She went from good teacher to miracle worker when she broke me of my worst habit when I was in the program. Eating next to nothing was standard on weigh in day. So, I'd be starving. This was followed by a gargantuan binge post class that often extended for days. It was my free day. I was attending in the evenings after work, so this was a long time with next to no food. It must have shown. I was listlessly waiting in line while she was mingled one by one down it. When she came to me, she said, 'You haven't eaten anything all day, have you?' I didn't even get a chance to reply before she went on. 'I know you haven't. You NEED to stop it!' Wow, the magic bullet hit me. I knew she was right. If it seems a no brainer to you, good readers, you need to re-examine it. Logic and addiction are often diametrically opposed. Smart people do ridiculously dumb things in the name of feeding the need. I ruined many a decent momentum with my 'starve and binge' syndrome. I was caught by Zelda and called on it and since she seemed to be right about everything else, why would this be different. I never had a 'free day' again.

Goal weight was around the corner when Zelda stuck a job application in my hand because I was going to work for the program. That was that. I hadn't really thought about it. But I was an obedient student and knew arguing was futile. So, I filled it out and gave it to her. It would change my life! Thank you, Zelda. At my final graduation with my mentor, Felicia, I was deeply touched when Zelda appeared there. I was not expecting her and nearly cried as she entered the room. My training director told me she was even more surprised. She'd skipped her own meetings to be there and she was evidently quite money driven. "She must REALLY like you", I was told. Zelda didn't witness the best meeting, but her presence touched me, deeply.

ICKY PART: Zelda also worked for another company and blended their business interests a lot in the classes. Her primary focus was always the program, but she did cross pollinate. Evidently, she'd been told not to do this repeatedly. She was fired. She had the better income from the other business, so I know she wasn't left hanging. But, the beginning of my professional life with the program did launch with my teacher being gone very soon after.

Many years later, I ran into her at a Starbucks. She recognized me, I recognized her voice. She had regained all her weight. It was awkward. My teacher that I credit with so much of my success had backslid. Considering that she'd been fired, it was understandable that she would not return to us for help. We exchanged a few words, said, 'So Long'. I wished I'd not run into her. I hoped she'd find her way back to the woman I'd met. From what I heard last (her sister has also been in and out of the program), that has not happened. But nothing will ever override what she did for me. My life was changed for the better by what happened to me in her classes. Lessons I cling to for strength to this day Zelda, bless you, again.

TIPS: Better eating needs to become your new lifestyle – Zelda walked it! I have followed that suit. Also, she risked telling people what they didn't want to hear at that moment. But it was what they needed to hear. I'd follow that example when I was counseling people, too. You need truth- sayers in your life.

TRAPS: Don't hurt yourself as a kneejerk reaction when someone hurts you. As I said, she'd been fired. But, regaining her weight did no one any good. Only Zelda carries it around again. You help nothing by harming yourself.

KEN:

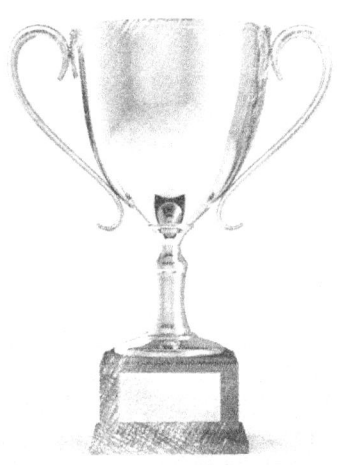

Ken walked in, filled out a registration form and joined the program for the first time. A Southern man with mischief in his eye and a keen sense of humor, I liked him and was glad he joined my class. Despite being of AARP age, he was an eternal young man. He listened to the details of how the program works and then, mysteriously, would not quite get the results at the scale. We'd talk and he would seem to hear my advice yet no difference in the outcome on weigh day. Hmmmm. What was the problem?

First of all, Ken's attendance was sporadic. We monitor our own member's records and I always look at my classes before time. This gives me an idea of what's going on with their progress and I can fine tune my mingle time with them. Receptionists are on the pulse of each person's weight and I need to be, too. Not every member shares their struggles and I can approach those members to offer help in a private way. Sometimes it's just what they need and they open up.

Being quiet was not a problem for Ken. He shared in his casual way and often made intelligent points with wit that charmed the members. Ken was an avid exerciser which made his lack of weight loss more frustrating. He was in great shape. My initial suspicion was that Ken was among the members I've encountered who rely too much on that good habit to the detriment of the necessary discipline regarding food. I found out later this was a correct hunch.

Ken would come and go from the program with a similar pattern: join - hey, good to have you back - let's do this - he works out like a mad man - no weight loss. I'd ask for his journals, make suggestions and not see the pattern change. A successful man, he was used to tackling projects and nailing them. This was not pleasing him that this wasn't happening this time. I respected his dedication to exercise and bent his ear for tips in that area. He proved very willing to share his time and a friendship began.

I am good at switching roles of student and teacher. Not everyone is good at this. In fact, when I auditioned to be a program teacher in an open call, there was a school teacher. I thought I was out of consideration. How could I compete? Turned out it was the fact that I wasn't a school teacher that impressed the training director. School teachers are often locked into an "I teach, you listen, itinerary driven" style she wasn't looking for. I was glad to be a blank slate to be molded.

Ken's personal stories of his own experiences were lively and I discovered there wasn't much Ken hadn't done in his life: travels, writing, military service, marksman, corporate business, entrepreneur, motorcycle enthusiast, computer whiz, photographer... I found it almost amusing as his list of accomplishments got longer with each luncheon or workout. We also could make each other laugh with a mutual wicked sense of humor. Ken was a good guy. I was determined to be of use to him regarding his weight.

Now, I dug deeper. Ken's personality was such that part of the weight loss journey would require some fundamental changes to his approach. He kept meticulous spread sheets and was detail oriented, as am I, but wasn't fully releasing his control to the program. Not giving 100%, well I had a master's degree in this. I have had to tell many members that the human body is not like a machine or a car. You can't say "If I do this and this and this I should logically see X results multiplied by X weeks." It isn't designed to work that way. Frustrating as that is, it's true. Ken liked being in control. He'd built a very impressive list of achievements with this method. I knew he needed to listen to me on this, but wasn't fully willing to. Ken would come and go a couple more times.

The second to last time, we worked together much closer. The daily weighing wasn't doing Ken any good. Nor was the lack of variety. The daily suggested food allotments - what daily food allotments, Ken often underrate and felt the disappointment when it didn't make the scale drop. I saw the binges followed by hellacious amounts of exercising. If this was a sample of a random member, I'd grade it a C.

Ken was as much a friend as I'd let any member become. I feel that it can muddle membership in the program. Relatives and people I've known many years have told me they intentionally did not join my class for that reason. I don't mind. Ken was also good at accepting the role of student when it was needed even though he was a teacher in many fields. He needed to find his exhaustion point in trying to lose his way as I'd had to. I took me 20+ years before I was willing to surrender, so Ken's few years, from our meeting to the present, was much quicker than mine.

He looked at my program, the foods I kept at home, how I ate out and knew my maintenance was in its 15th year. Something great happened - Ken told me he was going to reach out to me and follow the program under my guidance. His weight was getting in his way and this man of action didn't like feeling limited. Also, his workouts were very intense and to still be 60 or 70# overweight got under his skin, too. The guidance with how I track and shop was easy to share if a member is open to receive it. We went to the grocery store together, Ken used the same tracking methods I did (a computer ace, this old school approach I use was a good sign to me Ken was serious) and then worked on the concept of rearranging what he ate and when he ate. My unconventional meals may not be to everyone's taste, but I abide by them and they keep me thin and satisfied.

Well, Ken began losing weight. His next rejoining will be the one Ken makes goal with. His meticulous nature, intelligence and great exercising habits combined with the food program he's following will not fail him. Another success after 60, another success from the South, another success via tracking on paper, another success with the accountability of weekly class attendance, another success in a life with many successes under his belt. My friend Ken is a future goal achiever. Mark my word.

TIPS: Surrender to be taught. If you're a successful Type-A lone wolf, this can be difficult. Like me, Ken came to it only after extensive resistance. Believe this, teachable students willing to be taught benefit handsomely.

TRAPS: Fighting futility only drowns hope, drains energy and leads to dropping out of the battle. The human body is a strange and remarkable thing. See it for what its natural flow is and functions are and you'll prosper. Try to make water flow upstream and you'll die trying.

MONEY MATTERS:

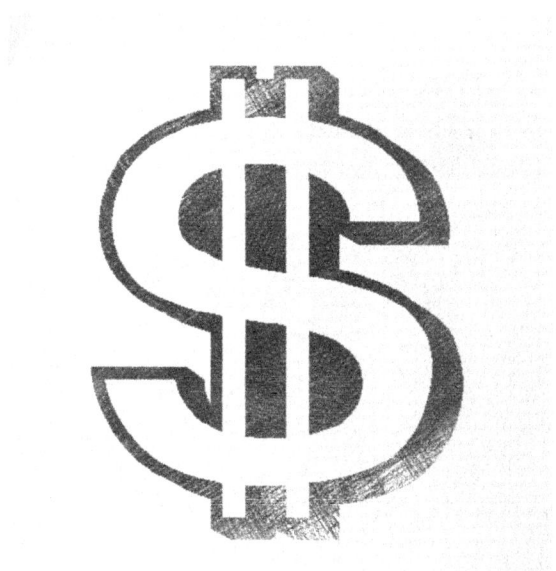

Money is the root of all evil. Money makes the world go around. Money can't buy happiness. Agree or disagree with those clichés. The program is a business. All businesses exist to provide a service via which they seek to make money. It's the essence of capitalism. There's nothing wrong with that. Most people have to work most of their lives and earn just enough money to get by. How it's spent is a private matter. I know that most of my life, the largest majority of my money went to food. Not survival food. I mean gluttony food.

I've never been rich. Not even upper middle class. A working Joe all my life, I've always been able to pay my bills. Not one to live extravagantly. That's the key to financial solvency. It's less to do with what you earn, it's what you spend! All this sound perspective has a point related to this book that'll make it seem topsy-turvy, indeed. But, it's my truth and many members I've met.

I consider over eating an addiction. No question about it. Just like you can be addicted to nicotine, alcohol, tobacco, all manner of drugs, glue sniffing.... I'm not factoring in the things we've accepted as addictions that are not literally physical addictions, i.e. —gambling, cheating on spouses, lying...Over eating is as much of an addiction as anything. It gets less sympathy and understanding than most others while its damage is broader than many other addictions. I don't understand what we don't understand. You cannot be addicted to eating, per se. Your body requires food for survival. Like the body requires sleep, breathing, eliminations. You CAN be addicted to over eating. I have been afflicted since my earliest memories and struggle with its pull daily.

Now that that has been established, back to money. Most addicts become very one dimensional people. Everything revolves around the addiction, its procurement, consumption and whatever means necessary to get money to keep the cycle going. This oh, so, sensible fellow in regards to money in all other aspects of his life has been on a continuous quest for food. Food isn't free. I don't live on a farm to grow it myself. I go to supermarkets, convenience stores, drive throughs, bakeries, restaurants, vending machines, mini bars, open markets, grocery stands, other people's houses and even, in my most desperate times, garbage cans for it. Back in the day, nothing got this lazy boy running quicker than the ice cream man. Excepting dumpsters and the occasional party - no one gave it away. It took money.

What's an addict (remember, compulsive over eaters are addicts) supposed to do when they're in the clutches of their substance? Lose distractions! What is a distraction? LIFE IS!!! Careers - distraction. Relationships - distraction. Friends - distraction. Hobbies - distraction. Exercising - (please, that was a joke) distraction. Doing your part to make the world a better place - unless patronizing many food establishments frequently enough that employees know your name and refer to your most often bought items as your 'usual' is doing my part - distraction. Religion - distraction. Politics - distraction. Kids - distraction. Vacations - distraction. Pretty much anything other than your addiction becomes a distraction. Spending money on things other than your addiction - sigh, distraction. This is identifiable to anyone who's ever sunk into the throes of addiction. Change the substance, you'll see your story in it.

So, when people join the program, they have to spend some money. They're set prices that I have no control over or negotiating room. When potential members try to haggle over fees, ask if there's a 2 for 1 discount, bring a friend rebate, etc. I inform them of this fact. We're not a used car lot or in a real estate transaction. Hemming and hawing being done, most join.

Then, the recommendations for a healthier lifestyle come at them. Balkers often justify their hesitation at the higher price that can accompany the suggested foods for better eating habits. Sociologists confirm that overweight and obesity hits economically lower middle class and the impoverished at a much higher rate than those above the middle class line. Junk food is cheaper. It's much cheaper. The lower the price tag, the unhealthier selections get.

There are same tools sold at program locations that make the journey easier. A food scale is very necessary. Trying to guess in their minds food portions is next to impossible. Most overweight people have completely out of whack ideas of the portions they're eating. But, it's $40+. Books with handy guidance for supermarket shopping and eating out are available to purchase. An electronic calculator that factors in nutrition is useful, too. Many members have squawked at this, too. As you delve deeper into rearranging your entire life, a gym membership or lessons for an activity may be due.

My best counter proposal has always been - what about the money you spent before you joined the program on food? You never cared then, did you? Not for a second, for most of us. When you were answering the door for the pizza delivery man, you couldn't toss the $20 bill at him quickly enough so you could start eating. Maybe even told him to keep the change as his tip, too! We've bought bags and bags of candy at Wal-Mart. Boxes and crates and mega sized jars of fattening items at volume markets that require private membership and provide numerous electric carts for the numerous obese shoppers. Restaurant meals in anyplace from fast food places, diners, buffets, family chains, cafes, mom and pop hole in the wall joints, fancy dining experiences - all ending with you leaving with a stuffed stomach and departing of some of your money - only talking about how yummy the food was, how full you are, how you liked or did not like the service.... the money? That's what money is for!

But, when I suggest it be spent on something that's going to benefit your life for a long time - WOO, do people resist. My 2nd effective counter proposal - pretend its food from before you were on the program. Spend it with the same abandon you did when it was doughnuts, French fries, chips, cookies, burgers, ribs, candy......you didn't look back. Also, when it was spent, the food eaten, it's gone. The only remnants are the damage. Damage like overweight, indigestion, bloating, gas, poor sleep, joint inflammation, sweat, clothes not fitting, guilt.... I could go on and on. Meanwhile, a food scale, measuring spoons are one time investments. I have broken through to many people this way.

It's a redefinition of what is cheap and what is expensive. The cost of the necessary things to get you thin and healthy is 1/2 dollar amount and 1/2 priceless.

TIPS: Log prices for a reality check for one month. See what you would have spent an excess food. It'll be a mindblower.

TRAPS: When I was new, I had a realization. On a hot summer day, I needed to do some errands. Go to the bank, pick up dry cleaning and buy stamps, very routine stuff. As I was about to leave, I realized I was not going to do these errands and eat. I stopped. I didn't want to go. I was as deflated as I could get. It was just too hot, anyway. Funny, when going to the bank, picking up dry cleaning and buying stamps included side trips for food, it wasn't too hot. Same principle applies to money distribution. Perspective!

WANDA:

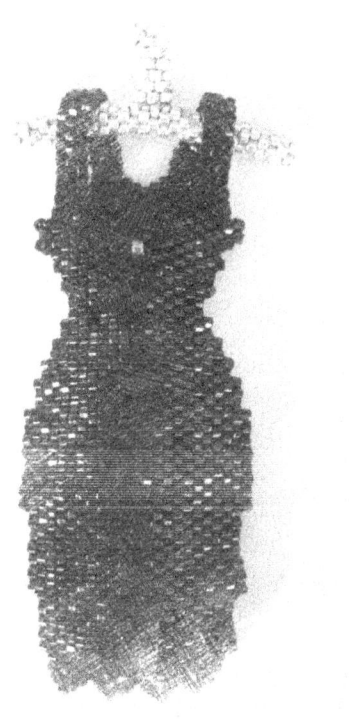

Wanda is a great example of what I admire so much about women. Women like her are the program's bread and butter: 35-55 years of age, life-long dieter, has a family whose needs overtook her taking care of herself and acknowledges that she needs our help. Women are much better at this. Men hold onto the 'lone wolf, I can do it alone' mentality more often. Asking for help is a sign of weakness and 'men aren't weak' or some other worn out rationale. Kudos to the 'real' men who join us, too! But, this isn't their story. Women seek out the community meeting atmosphere and nurture it.

Wanda was 40-something and had both personality and style. She spoke with authority and heart (a great combination - she could do anything). I liked her from the jump. Wanda was stylishly groomed. Hair, make up, nails, outfit, shoes were all on point. When I see overweight people that just let themselves go, I wonder when they reached the point where they felt it was pointless to even try to put any effort into their appearance. After all, look how big they are, right? WRONG! In fact, you should put more effort into it. It keeps your self-esteem pilot light on. Dimly, perhaps, but ON! I am the electrician whom members look to to have theirs stoked or reignited. I care and I want them to care, too!

Wanda obviously cared. So, off we went. 70# to lose, I'd say. As the program began, Wanda opened up about her food obsessed upbringing that put her on this path - got it. A busy lifestyle with children, a job, a home and obligations that distracted her from the fact that the years were passing and her weight was getting in the way of everything - got it. Wanda also had a husband uninterested in healthy eating and not on board with this endeavor - sigh, got it.

Granted, there are always 2 sides to any story, but I've heard this too often to doubt it. A very common domestic snag in so many ladies' battle to rearrange her food life and bring about the change she desires: the husband. Wanda's is Italian —so I must understand that they EAT, they only cook ONE WAV, they don't like CHANGE, they're STUBBORN, they won't allow the program's eating plan to permeate their meals, so there must be 2 meals made for family

PEACE. Girl, please! As a man, let me clue you into something. Do you know why so many men pull this? <u>Because you keep letting them get away with it.</u> Yes, ladies. YOU play a part in this unbalanced, unfair and ridiculous play. End Scene!

Wanda had her work cut out for her, but she had a strong will that she was going to rediscover and use now. She took to the common sense and flexibility of the program well. Also, Wanda bought into the good tasting recipes and began experimenting with them. To her delight and surprise, they were mostly very good and didn't require much extra work. This made her daily routine less of an obstacle and onward she went. Her losses each week seemed to bring in a different woman the next week. She shared how each new meal went over primarily at home, but also when she ate out and when she was at social functions. How easy this was! Wanda kept my advice close at hand regarding meal changes at home with less than cooperative spouses. Don't say anything. Most often resistance is mental and if you say nothing, they'll eat it without the 'Eww, it's diet food. I won't like it.' close mindedness. This was working. Her kids, friends and even her husband ate many adjusted dishes without mentioning a word - unless it was to compliment it.

As months went by, the weight loss seemed to raise Wanda's spirit, commitment, skirt hem and heels. This lady exuded confidence and it became her. She knew she was looking good and why shouldn't she feel great about that! She'd comment on how other ladies at her kids' schools gawked as she picked them up - easily the most glamorous mama in the room at 3:30pm! The most encouraging part was that this was happening without feeling deprived or struggling with having to accept a life of bland food, difficult daily altering of a schedule, prohibitive exercising regimens.... none of that: just the program.

While it would be nice to say hubby enjoyed this new wife of his enough to change his ways, real life isn't like fairy tales- Wanda went to the gym, weight loss classes, journaled her food, got online info regarding dining out, tried new recipes all while having to make traditional, fattening tempting dishes for him: twice the work, cleaning up.... not to mention the morale deflation of living with someone so unwilling to offer up any sort of help regarding such an important thing. I suggested many times she have a talk with him, I also invited him to come to a class to see what we do so it wasn't a big secret.... no, no. He was what he was and outside of divorce, it was on her to accomplish this in that situation. Could Wanda keep strong?

Yes, she could. A vacation without a weight gain seemed especially empowering for her. They'd always been a waterloo of pounds in the past and she wasn't as sure of herself. Not only did she rise to the occasion, she had a taste of what travelling could be without food as the sole focus. She walked, played, took pictures, bought clothes, calmly ate her way and let others eat theirs. She was still on the dazzled euphoria of this at her next weigh in. She could do anything, now.

Including shop! Wanda was looking hotter than ever. Buying clothes was emerging as her favorite past time. She found the 'I can walk into any store and know they'll have my size' so darn joyful it added rocket fuel to her will power. If she'd given up the way she used to eat, she had to have a substantial reward to take its place, right? Right! Clothes, it was! Wanda was the thinnest, most attractive of all her middle school kids' parents. She felt tremendous. Life as a thin person was the one she'd live.

Wanda is a model for any woman - or man, really - to aspire to. She's bought into the program for life, still at goal, looking great, smiling easily and genuinely whenever I see her, still attached to the husband that never got on board with this and still someone I'm sure has cracked this code forever. She is a heroine!

TIPS: Revel in your success! Wanda lives this to the hilt! If you make sacrifices, what are they for? Deny yourself the rewards and spoils, you deny joy. The work will likely be abandoned one day.

TRAPS: Wanda's strong, strong will isn't common. Making 2 meals to accommodate un- cooperative spouses won't garner sympathy or support. Risk talking to them, you know the right words. If they get 100% away with never having to help, they won't. Maybe full throttle help won't happen, but nothing comes from nothing.

PENNY:

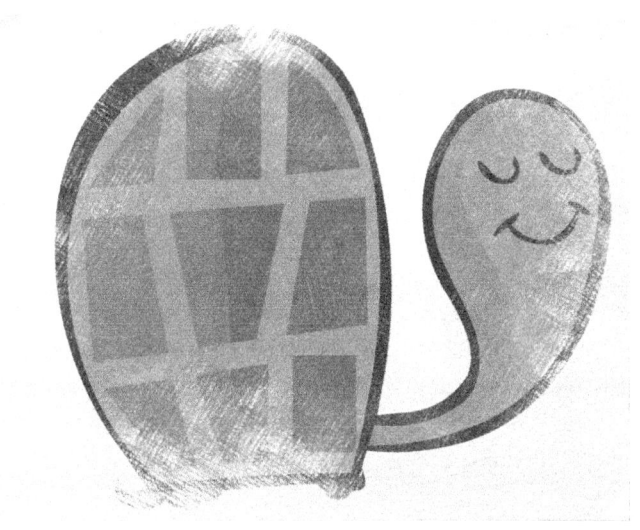

The program meeting facilities sometimes keep before and after photos of members. Not all of them do. I don't know why. It's so impressive as a business move, if nothing else, for prospective joiners to see. Also, current members struggling can look at others who've been right where they are and kept going. You might only have a brief moment to inspire someone to not quit when they're at a breaking point. At that moment, I think those pictures do this far better than any words I know. Enter Penny.

I've pointed her photos out to members many times and for good reason. Penny had many obstacles most of us won't endure and didn't allow them to dictate her future. When they hear me explain it after they've SEEN her photos, they often walk away motivated to keep working towards their own goals. The photo snagged them in and I seal the deal by explaining the story behind it - another member doesn't quit. If you believe in positive karma, then Penny continues to accumulate it year in and year out.

Superficial challenges first: Penny was over 60 and had given up since she'd bought into the fable that it was too late. Penny was 80+# overweight and nothing had ever worked and she'd bought into the fable that she was a hopeless case. Penny was from the South and 'they fry everything' and she'd bought into the fable that it was 'cultural and natural' for her to eat this way. Penny was from an obese family and bought into the fable that it was genetic that they were all big. Not massive overeaters, it was genetic.

Deeper challenges: Penny had rheumatoid arthritis. A lousy disease: very lousy. It doesn't kill you, but it keeps you in pain for years. You need to take medicines that will have significant side effects limiting your mobility, energy level and affect your weight. Or you can live with pain. This is a choice? Penny had diabetes in her family and blood pressure meds and insulin were on the horizon among possible surgeries for joints succumbing to the RA. Also, organ damage is a 'side effect' of the meds. Penny was on a steroid regimen that made her body reluctant to give up the pounds no matter what she did. Most challenging of all: Penny had 99% given up on herself when I met her. I am so glad she took to the program before the final 1% closed her off to an unhappy forever after.

Penny's meds, as I'd said, made it very rough for her to lose weight. It wouldn't be impossible, but very hard. Steroidal meds blew her body up, made her metabolism sluggish to say the least and sometimes bloated her hands to the point where driving was difficult. I had to spend extra time with her because her case was much more intense than the typical member. She needed customizing to her program and pep talks to keep her going. I was glad to give both.

Her body: I had to tell her the things she may not have wanted to hear, but I knew she needed to know. Realistic expectations for Penny were that her margin for error was about nil. Who among you reading this would want to be told that? I also used the new (for me) tools called the Internet to look up information on the many specific meds she was on to keep us both facile on what to expect next. Also, I prodded Penny to stay on her doctor's case about what she was taking, how much was vital, when could she take less, would weight loss make some of them unnecessary? Penny was like a puppy when their eyes open in this regard. She'd been of the generation that didn't question physicians. They were semi-Gods with diplomas and she was just a 'small town Southern girl' and who was she to say anything but 'yes' – wrong! It raised Penny's morale to participate in her own recovery (a phrase I LOVE!). I am glad her physicians took to their new patient. She became more aware of her own diagnosis' than she'd been her entire life. She could look forward to coming down or entirely off some meds if she lost weight. POWER!!

Her morale: Penny was not able to make even the slightest lee way and expect to lose weight. This was the card she'd been dealt. So, while it was physically possible - how to keep her focused and believing her goal was doable? Penny definitely needed someone to believe in her. I was glad to be that true fan for her. To make it rougher, Penny's reward for the perfect program she'd need to uphold would be min-iscule losses or no losses at all sometimes. Mercy! No wonder Penny had succumbed to the mountain of discouraging prognosis and led the grim life of an obese, aged before her time woman. I locked into the zone with Penny by assuring her that the double length it would take would not be her undoing. The same amount of time would pass whether she did this or not. If I said it will take 4 years, why not do this? It will be 4 years from now either way. This seemed to light a fire in Penny and I knew she would be alright. When I see the fire in a person, they're usually going to make it. This simple piece of logic had slipped under the radar for Penny. It does for many people.

No one in her family was bothered by Penny's poor health. This did her no favors. Seeing her lose weight without support made her class time truly a life line. She shared weekly and inspired many with her amazing strength, good attitude and lack of bitterness over her difficult road. Penny was still Southern. Fried food was a big temptation that she had to fight daily. Subtle changes in her eating regimen suited her. It seemed no one noticed the salads she was making and eating with the beige carb glut fests that were her family meals. Why say anything? They'd only dump on it in between gobs of gravy soaked, artery clogging glop and make her feel bad. Who needs that?

Seemed that thinking about Penny's needs was not something she was used to and, boy, she liked it. With time, the weight came off at a snail's pace. She'd gripe when her perfect adherence to the program had yielded zero loss at the scale. She needed to vent and I'd let her get it all out before I'd come at her with any offers of advice. We all need to just vent and talk about it without immediate fix it ideas sometimes. The next week, she'd be in smaller clothes (corduroy slacks were of particular joy for her - a milestone) and her smile would be as wide as her face again.

When Penny made goal, it took less than 4 years. It had taken 3 and ½. She'd done it. With an after picture that was a mouth dropping contrast to the before one. That lady didn't exist anymore. The extra jowls, double chin, dowdy clothed, gray haired very old looking woman in her late 50s had been shed. In her place was a cheek boned, green and red striped sweater (size M) over tan cords, boots (!) wearing woman with a modern hair cut in her early 60s! Penny still had RA. She'd accomplished this with a list of potential obstacles that would have overwhelmed many people to never try and she did it. When her husband retired and they moved away, we embraced over 'so longs' and tears. My faith in her will never waver.

Her photos still inspire people many years later.

TIPS: Patience is required of all of us, but Penny had it in spades. The concept of disregarding a schedule or deadlines proved freeing. Think of your last 3,4 or 5 diets you've quit. Do you remember why you quit? Do you realize if you hadn't, you could be thin right now? Doesn't the reason you quit seem silly now compared to that? Penny had a plan!

TRAPS: Penny faced an obstacle course of 'em. Don't be reluctant to question doctors. It's your body. Also, there is no predestination to your obesity. Do not fall into that trap. It's not 'in your blood', it's 'on your plate.'

WILLIAM:

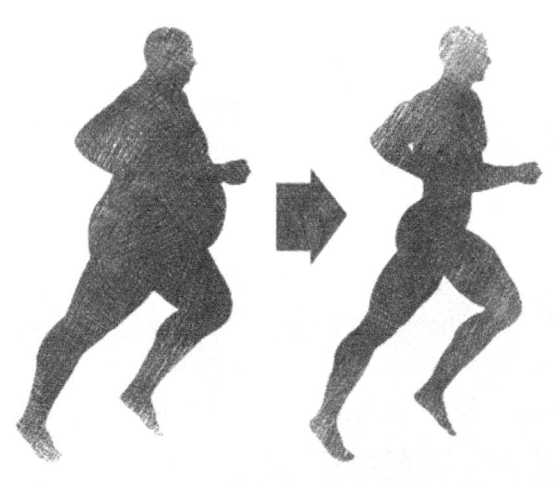

William joined the program with his wife. They were both considerably overweight, but very congenial. Athletic and not obese in his youth, he seemed to say that marriage was fattening without actually saying it. I've come across this often. When 2 people marry or live together, they take on each other's habits. Getting into a rut of overeating and not being active happens too often in this blissful security. Ironically, it also often is the cause of that very blissful secure environment becoming unstable.

William and his wife were not unhappy with each other. Their love was obvious, but they were far too young to be as heavy as they were and it was affecting their lives in many negative ways. Time was not going to wait for them. William's problems were typical. Prone to over-doing most of his eating, he was lax to non-existent in portion control. Simply put, William would eat until he was full! Uncomfortably full. Satisfied was not a word used in his eating vocabulary. William relied on the most overused of clichés to justify it. He was older (in his 30s—ha!), he was a man and they have bigger appetites (maybe true to a point, but not to the tune of 80+# overweight), he was too busy to exercise (he'd been, among other things, an enthusiastic dirt bike rider, but he'd had to give it up because of his size) and, best of all, he was 'big boned'.

I wanna run with that one. Big boned is a highly relied on excuse men use for being overweight. Your skeletal bone structure is not in your control. This is true. But it's not a pre destiny for obesity or permission to eat oneself into oblivion. Big boned is a long, long stretch to double chins, bulging guts, tree trunk thighs and male breasts. No bone structure did any of that. Simply put, it's fat. But, we all want to take refuge in comfortable denials that enable us to continue on our destructive paths.

William had dreams and desires he'd kept quiet about. Personal reasons, I'm not sure about. But, I do identify with the secretive nature. Overweight people are so compromised in the options for what to do with their lives that a secret fantasy list of what we'd like to do 'if only I could lose the weight' is a common pipe dream we invest in. If they're particularly exciting or rely on beauty or physiques, we're even quieter about it. How can you talk about harboring a desire to dance if you're obese? Or dive? Or ride horses? Or zip line? Or kayak? Or ride hot air balloons? Or be a model, actor or rock star? The list is endless. These become heart locked desires we bury with food and accept that they'll never happen. That sucks.

Next phase is to ignore it. William was through with that. His dreams included getting back on the dirt bikes he loved. Dirt biking is not for the faint hearted. It's wild, dirty, risky and only for the adrenaline rush seekers. As William got heavier, it became impossible. A big reality 'ouch' moment came at one of his last times on a bike. Like I'd said, it's not for the timid. The younger guys often look at the seasoned guys for the thrill, to applaud them and learn tips. When William was done riding, he already knew he was not as able to tear up the course as he'd been. His weight kept the bike from handling curves or jumps. Also, he couldn't get the height or speed that makes the whole thing the thrill it should be. Adding insult to injury, when he finished one of his last rides, he realized the other guys were laughing at him: the 'fat guy on a bike - hysterical like a clown at a circus', his time there as a participant was over. Going to dirt bike trails and watching other guys ride wasn't his idea of fun. So, he put it behind him. Like most overweight people eventually have to do with their dreams. We eat them away.

William and his wife adopted a child. Having kids changes everything. Now, there weren't two obese adults living together. There was a baby. As is often the game changing move for new parents, it gave William a purpose and drive that he didn't have on his own. He knew he could not be the father he wanted to be at his size. There was so much he wanted to do with his son. Run with him, throw a ball, swim with him, fly kites, play horsey, ride rides in parks and so much more. His weight had to go, - NOW - back on program. William became a model student. He listened in class. He gave it his best efforts. He shared in meetings. He was obviously motivated and practiced the program. He impressed me and the class with his willingness to talk about how he had to invest in the entire program. Not only do the parts he found easy and convenient. This was what had always undone any previous diet he'd ever tried. Not being 100%.

Boy, did I understand that one. That was my standard for any diet. Give it a certain amount of effort and if that isn't enough, move on to the next one. Thinking there was some diet out there where 60% would do.

As the weight came off, William concentrated on exercising as well so that he wouldn't have the sagging skin problem people who take off as much weight as he was going to can encounter. The fire that was lit in him was reigniting not only his old jock with a heart confidence, but it opened up new vistas of what he may be capable of, too. Yes, he wanted to get back on the dirt bikes, but injury prone risks were not the stuff for new dads. William wanted to take up muscle building. Not just be 'fit enough for his age'. Apparently, he'd harbored interest in taking his body to its maximum potential for years, but kept it to himself. Like I'd said earlier, how can a 300+# man talk about his dream of being ripped and shredded without it seeming either comical or pathetic? It was his secret.

Not anymore. As William got closer to goal, he was concerned about maintenance because he was unsure what a proper direction would be for him since he wasn't entirely sure where the bouncing ball would settle. We would cross that bridge later. I didn't want this to become a distraction unnecessarily. First, get to goal. On the night William achieved this, his wife and baby lead the applause he richly deserved. When William spoke, he said something I've never forgotten and have repeated ever since. "I used to say I was big boned. I hid behind that for many years. I'm not big boned. As you can see, I'm average built." Nothing more needed to be said. It was perfect, true and very insightful. SO many men use that phrase to stay cocooned in denial and get diabetes, heart failure, joint pain, gout, high blood pressure and a myriad of other maladies that got their start in 'I'm big boned' rationalizing. He had an average physique. Who knew… shock and a half. I, too, am average physiqued. Not big, not skinny, but average.

As tears went down William's face, he looked at his child and said he knew he'd stay slim to provide the happiest childhood he could by being the best father he could. A fortunate kid, that is. I know William will make good on that promise. His tenacity will see him through. He is another of my hero's.

TIPS: If you're unsure about final figures because it's territory you've never been in, ask for guidance. William did and has had a much smoother time because of it.

TRAPS: William was a trap buster! Examine what clichés you're allowing to trap you (Williams' 'I'm big boned', 'we're curvy', 'I'm a good person underneath, it shouldn't matter') and euthanize them.

MISERY LOVES COMPANY:

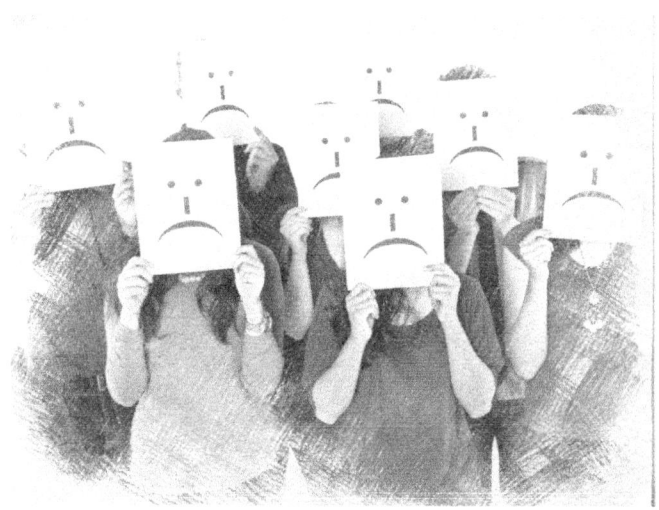

Here's an often played out scenario. Many times couples join together - WONDERFUL! Many men are reluctant to join. Feeling it's for women, their butch assuredness goes into panic mode. I get it. It takes a secure man, worthy of admiration. They seem to have the odds in their favor. Women attempt weight loss in greater numbers. Men join less, but those that do have a higher success rate, percentage wise.

Together or not, I hear many lady members lament the need for their husband or boyfriends or significant other to join, but it'll never happen. I leave that alone, usually. A wise instructor picks their battles thoughtfully. The male body is comprised of more fat burning muscle, so they have a leg up in weight loss. It's usually faster and easier. Yes, men are lucky. Any wise man will freely admit it. How many gray haired, potbellied, wrinkled women were ever considered 'somehow still attractive? Unfair! But, fair schmair, life isn't fair, so....

I've watched men lose weight while their lady sulked in a puddle of jealousy (men lose weight so much easier), resentment (I'm the one who got him to join!) or misguided competition (I was even heavier than he was and he STILL lost more!). Message to Matilda: You're not a man. Don't expect what Mother Nature's designed you to not do. Also, negative self- talk is unproductive. I've even seen couples quit over this or open sabotage. People do crazy things when they're in pain. Things they wouldn't do in any other situations but weight loss.

However, I have also seen more than a few ladies take another per- spective. I've watched women watching their man shed pounds which elicited praise for him, thus making her look worse by comparison. "What's he doing with her?" I cannot understand everything that goes on in a woman's head. I have a higher degree of understanding than most men. Some scenarios are universal, but some are not. So, please understand, dear reader, much of this is pure observation and openly expressed occurrences I've been privy to....

I quote directly, 'I'm not going to be 's fat wife!" Suddenly, the lady catches fire and runs with it. You look bigger by comparison if your mate is thin and you're not. When we're both heavy, it's more tol- erable. Of course, you should want to lose weight for personal rea- sons, such as improved health, better self-esteem, looks.... but if your spouse is also an overweight, couch potato, somehow we feel better. I've tried to imbue my wisdom, care, motivational speaking skills, compassion, nutrition ideas and experience and patiently heard excuses and nodded my head and bit my tongue over and over hoping I'll eventually break through and POW! Big mama's DOING it! Not by anything I did. No, her husband got thinner and so she did. The sole source of this fire was <u>not being 's fat wife'</u>. I'm not a fan of that being one's primary reason, but, hey, whatever works, right?

Well, not really. What happens when he falls off the wagon if that's your dangling carrot? Right, you fall with it. Oh, and don't forget, women are often very competitive with other women, too. It's a different version of the same game with some variations on the rules. If my sister, friend, cousin gets thin, I will be 's fat sister, friend, cousin and THAT gets 'em movin'! Try to have better motivation.

Overweight IS the final completely acceptable prejudice. The stigma is still allowed. Even if you privately hold tremendous hatred for certain people due to their race, religion, sexual orientation, gender.... you know the rules are pretty clear that you keep that kind of thinking private (or shared only in other likeminded company). But, it's still alright to make fun of fat people. You can tell jokes in work break rooms about them without worry about being in your boss' office being reprimanded. The sense of shame tied to being overweight keeps many from complaining. Comics still tell 'fat jokes' and no one seems to mind. You know it's true: Words hurt worse than weapons. It's unfair and needs to end. Maybe that makes folks who lose their weight with the program the best kind of thin person: compassionate ones, non-judgmental about those who still suffer. I have been thin many years and I still recall the scars, mocking, painful, day to day way of life in its many negative aspects. I'll never forget it. It keeps me focused on maintaining my program. But, I embrace every overweight person brave enough to walk in the door, dust themselves off and get on the horse again. It's never too late until you breathe your final breath.

TIPS: There's a positive productive way to use competition. If you're not going to be the bigger spouse, friend, sibling and it leads you to good healing behavior - go for it.

TRAPS: There's a negative unproductive side to this. The more personal and internal your motivation is, the steadier it is. Only one person on the entire planet can't say that they're now thinner than someone else. Aim higher.

DIANE AND HER EXCUSES:

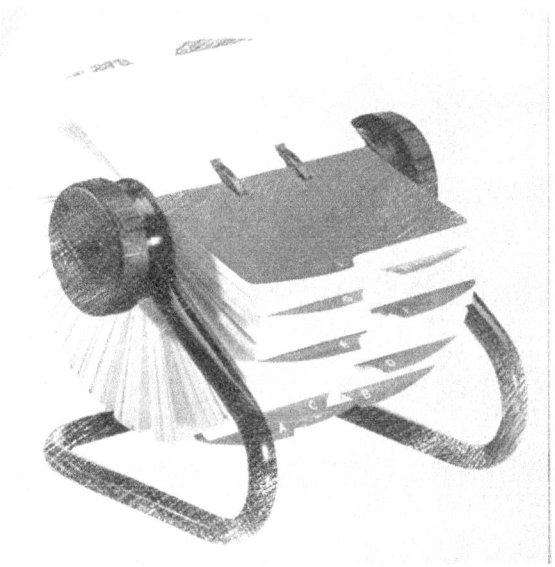

Excuses: I've told many of them through the years, the reasons why it was perfectly understandable that I didn't lose weight that week. Let's see, spin the wheel...'I had a bad week' (whatever that can mean - but, it's kind of ambiguous, so it doesn't elicit too many objections) —'I had to, bought it, baked it, made it and I couldn't hurt their feelings' - HA, that was a big lie. No one had their food eaten out of pity by me! I gobbled up massive amounts of food on a day to day basis no matter the source. 'It _____ day' - any and all holidays were a 100% glut fest with no questions. I could go on and on. Sound familiar? I had bad weather blamed, political elections, sport events, even 9/11.

No one ever directly called me on them. I don't believe I was done a favor by this. If I'd been challenged on them, I'd have had to explain them or justify them logically or be told I wasn't fooling them, at least. Perhaps I'd have thought twice before I tried stretching the truth so regularly.

WELL, my karma came when I became a full time weight loss counselor. Now, I am on the receiving end of excuses and am not a willing participant in the 'yea, ok, I'm buying this' part of the two-way charade. It's not that I have no understanding or compassion for those still suffering: far from it. It's <u>because </u>of that that I cannot enable people to continue letting years pass by while they sing the same worn out song. Not everyone is grateful for this honesty. I have had same express this by not returning to my class - keep searching for a teacher until they find one that says what they want to hear, yea, I've done that one, too. Others get wide eyed and look visibly shaken - THAT'S when I see an opening that I might dispense caring guidance that could break through and change their life! When the member has their eyes, ears, mind and heart open for new information, breakthroughs become reality!

Diane: Very timid soul. Barely spoke above a whisper. Shy is an understatement. But, she seemed to take to 'out there, loud, expressive me.' She was always willing to chat about her dilemmas one on one, but always clammed up in class. While I cannot privately council all members, I do it often when I feel there is a chance the member is only reachable this route and I feel a connection with them. Diane was such a case: petite mother of young children. She'd hit a wall and seemed unable to progress. It's a frustrating place to be. I've been there. But when I offered her good tried and true advice, somehow next week there was always a reason it didn't happen. A sick kid, a trip to Disneyland, lost her journal (because pens and paper are not easily gotten in America, that's a real problem) .... yet, I knew I had a responsibility to persevere with Diane. I felt if I didn't continue with her, she wouldn't extend herself again. So, we'd go on. I was patient with her, listened closely and always offered suggestions tailored to her. Exercise was not her favorite thing, as it is not for many over-weight people. The excuses were tossed at me like a Vegas black jack dealer (we can't afford it, I don't like crowds— so no classes or gyms, I'm too self-conscious to participate in group activities, kids need me to make lunch, do homework, sew...) I mean, she was committed to not move more.

But, she slipped up one week. She walked her small kids to school and home. I said she could make this her walking time. Quickly, she parried that the pace would be too fast for her children. I countered with she could walk briskly on the 1/2 of the walk she was alone: on the way home in the morning and on the way to school in the after-noon. POW! Since she seemed open and willing, I drove it further, suggesting she could walk up and down familiar streets thus extend-ing the walk for maximum benefit!

She was nonplussed and I just wore her down and she accepted this. It was also a time I took a chance and mentioned how great her walls of excuses were. She admitted it and told this was why she pursued me. I was good for her. Not to be confused with liked me. I have been told this many times. I will never be voted Miss Congeniality. There are teachers much more liked by their membership in an 'I'd invite her over for dinner' way. I don't need that, anyway. I have my own family and friends. Diane had the biggest losses she'd had in 7 months for the next few months. Diane had to move away before she'd made goal, but if she kept the habits she was on in the new state, I'm very confident she did just that!

Re-examine your excuses. Are you trying to justify non-efforts? If so, your reward is no progress. That's not going to do. Life won't wait. Please, end your relationship with them. If Diane could, you can, too!

TIPS: Look for 'can' at every opportunity, not 'cannot'. 99% of all cases, 'can' exists. Annihilate 'cannot'. Reach out to those who'll do you the most good. They don't have to be a friend.

TRAPS: It took weeks and weeks of one on one time to break Diane of her excuse pattern. You won't always have that to rely on. Nurture good habits regularly.

INGRID:

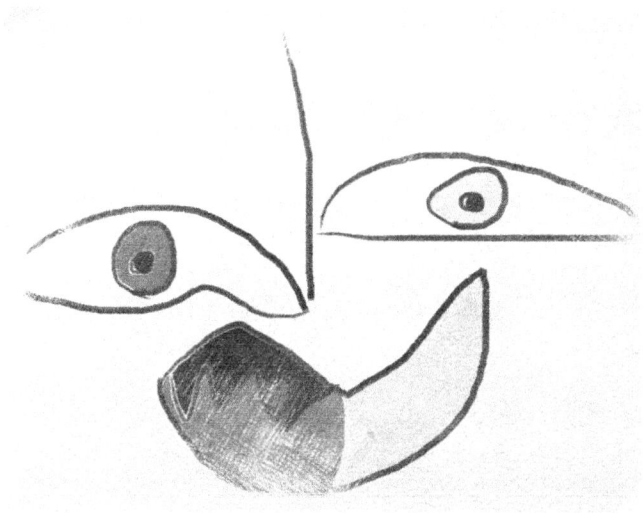

If Sesame Street's Oscar the Grouch had a mother, it might have been Ingrid. Ingrid walked in from the beginning with a grimace and never seemed to be having a good day, no matter what. Granted, I don't know the inner details of people's lives. As they open up, I'm offered access to personal information that helps explain their destructive relationship with food. So, giving Ingrid the big benefit of the doubt, I tried the 'shine it on' approach. I believe it's wise both on a personal and professional level. Ingrid was very short, over 70 years old and about 30# overweight. It irked her - this extra weight. I liked that it irked her. Irked means she cared. It's vital to be profoundly dissatisfied with where you are to make any genuine effort to change. The ones that are complacent or too accepting of their state are far less likely to see much happen. At 4'11", this extra weight was enough to be concerned about. At Ingrid's age, it was definitely something to be concerned about. With her health on the line, we locked arms together.

Sounds chummier than it was. Ingrid didn't drive anymore and came on the senior transportation van. They never seemed to be doing their job right, either. Most people didn't seem to do their job right for Ingrid. I'd get her weekly sneer while I tried my best to act happy to see her. Strangely, I was happy to see her. Usually, negative people are to be avoided like poison ivy in my book. But, this was different, this was in a work related atmosphere and because I did sense the willingness to follow the program correctly in Ingrid.

Being old school suited us as pilot and co-pilot. She wrote her food down and believed computers were inventions of the devil. She liked the supermarket and dining out guides we sell and used them thoroughly. Her biggest dilemma was with the dining commons and their preparation. Oh, I'd neglected to mention earlier, Ingrid lived in a senior retirement facility where they weren't doing their jobs to Ingrid's satisfaction, either. Ingrid did NOT cook (another grunt and sneer shot at me when I brought it up). Ingrid ate what they provided. I assumed that in a place with all senior residents would be very used to and prepared for dietary needs. Things like diabetes, allergies, weight loss and many other varying factors would make a varied menu necessary. Not so, Ingrid said. In fact, the place served crappy greasy food she'd never have eaten in her own home. For proof, she brought in the weekly menus. Ingrid was right. The gravies, white bread, fried options, desserts, whole milk, processed foods were the majority of what I saw. This wouldn't do.

Now, I was irked. Ingrid had to subside on their food. We had a project to tackle. I needed her to discuss her food alterations she'd require with the facility manager, but she didn't know exactly what do ask. That was my specialty. I combed the menus and wrote the questions I had about the entrees, sides, salads and desserts on post-it notes so Ingrid could go back and find out what they were really using and what could be changed. I smiled as I thought of the poor people who said 'no' to Ingrid.

We'd whittle at the menu and I do admit we saw progress. Ingrid lost weight pretty regularly. She liked these jelly like candies we sell that seemed to tickle her taste buds that I find repugnant.

Interestingly, lots of seniors like them. Maybe I will one day, too. Ingrid had a lot going for her. Tenacity and being assertive are a good one - two combo and Ingrid socked it to them every week armed with what I gave her. Sometimes, we really had to wing it. She said the portions were too much since the servers tended to plop the stuff on. Just like any cafeteria I've ever been in. Why do they all do that? Is it something they train? Use of her little hands as guidelines could manage that well enough.

Ingrid loved to exercise. That was her other secret weapon. I was very impressed by how much she liked it. I have so many people who use their age as an excuse for why they cannot. I meet many inspired and inspiring seniors who put them to shame with their dedication. I can 'go there' with these folks because my generation, (40 / 50 somethings) are the biggest excuse makers on this one. Ingrid would get in the senior transportation van daily for the ride to wherever they worked out. The thought of Ingrid in leotards, bright sneakers and a bandana lifting weights made me have to stifle laughs in class when she talked about lt.

Ingrid didn't take not getting what she wanted well. No, she didn't. If Ingrid gained, would I hear about it. A quarter pound up would be treated like a 4-month long plateau that defied explanation. Foolishly, I tried logical rational talking with Ingrid, at first. Results – Zilch! Ingrid had to vent, I know, she needed to vent about nearly everything - to me. Gains are a part of the weight loss game. Granted, they're not the fun part, but they are a part of it. This did very little to appease Ingrid. I would think I'd talked her down, then in the meeting I'd ask if anyone had a question and Ingrid would say, 'How can I possibly have gained this week?' Didn't we just talk about this? Thankfully, Ingrid attended a small meeting. She required a lot of extra time. This I had to give. If she were in a busier class, that would not have been possible.

The 'Ingrid didn't take not getting what she wanted well' I said in the last paragraph really was true. She changed convalescent homes. They just weren't up to scratch. 'Wow, Ingrid, really, you moved?' I said. "Yea, I got sick of them not listening to me and being late picking me up and serving all that crap." I hope I stand up for myself if I'm in Ingrid's place at that age. Maybe I'll be a bit nicer about it. Oh, well, change of locale, but the game remains the same.

Ingrid made goal and when she did, she actually smiled. It was scary. I thought it was an evil set up. She was quite proud of herself and deservedly so, but, Ingrid didn't smile. Well, it didn't last. I should have taken a photo -just wait. When people get to goal, they're always offered the chance to get up and talk to the class. Ingrid wanted her moment. After the applause stopped, tiny little Ingrid in her blue jogging suit (either she bad a closet of this same jogging suit or nothing else at all) went off: "I'M 77 YEARS OLD! I LOST THIS WEIGHT! I'M TIRED OF HEARING PEOPLE SAY HOW HARD IT IS! IT'S WORK! I GET UP EVERY DAY and I EXERCISE! I RUN! I LIFT WEIGHTS! I SWIM! I WATCH WHAT I EAT! I TRACK! NO SITTING ON MY DUFF (a word no one under 70 says)! JUST GET UP and DO THIS! Oh, and, (glance my way) you're the best." Then she sat down.

Ingrid's tongue lashing done, no one clapped due to the dressing down they'd all received by a thin older lady that really was saying mostly 100% true words. But, Ingrid, delivery is everything. Her compliment to me was about as sweet as Ingrid would get. Sigh, a change in schedule forced Ingrid and I to say 'so long'. She had no family and no friends (wonder why) to drive her to the program center. I know she will do well on her own. Very few do, but I know Ingrid will. Why? Because the last thing she told me before leaving was that while we'd been working on her food and weight loss, she'd been taking basic computer skills classes and would continue online. Wow, Ingrid.

Wow.

TIPS: Bypass menus if they don't meet your needs. If you have to ask, then ask. Exercise is so crucial to keep you healthy as you age. If it isn't given up, it doesn't have to be restarted!

TRAPS: Be nice. More people are attracted to honey than vinegar. Why I felt close to Ingrid, I can't fully explain. Don't look to angel interventions too often.

KEVIN:

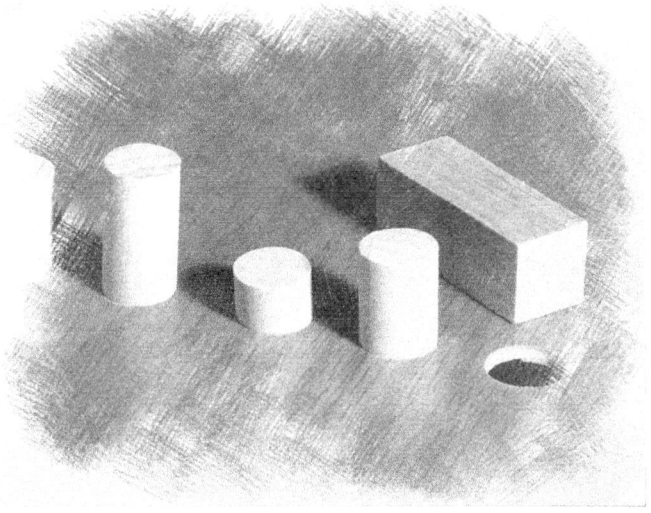

Kevin was a skeptic. He came to his first meeting with a 'show me' chip on his shoulder. I have met this type many times. Rookies often join the program doubting it'll work for them. The reasons: people have failed on diets many times, they're tentative to get their hopes up, they view the programs' stellar reputation with ambivalence and the classes are what they're not looking forward to. Whatever Kevin may have had in his head; it was a scowl on his face that I got. He didn't want to be there. But, he had family involvement. His daughter in law and her parents joined with him. This support system can be great. But, if one is dragooned into a project as personal and labor intensive as the program against their will, that doesn't work. The other 3 folks he signed up with were as opposite to him as could be: smiling, perky, enthusiastic, seemed full of faith. I don't pick the members. I open the door and we take it from there.

But, I can say I give them all my best. They expect my best. Deserve my dedication. They need to be listened to and they need to HEAR. In his late 50s with a good 70# too much, Kevin laid his money down. He may not realize how much he benefitted from the environment he launched in. The testimonials came weekly from the other members of his troop that the program was being embraced, followed carefully and the results were obvious at the scale. His daughter in law was a sweet young lady. She blossomed and it seemed to have a warming effect on Kevin. He mellowed somewhat as he reaped the rewards eating healthy gives. When the skeptic allows the program to work, their state of mind can improve. Physical pain makes people angry. They can even show resentment to those trying to help them. Being relieved of the pain was transforming Kevin for the better. He kept his salty exterior, but I could see he was glad to be there. Well, glad could be a stretch, but he met my eyes when I greeted him and the corners of his mouth turned upwards. I'll take it.

As a team, all 4 of them made goal. Between them, it was somewhere in the 200+# range. Magnificent! Glorious! A stellar success! Kevin took off 70# and talked openly in meetings about the changes he made in his day to day life and in his attitude. He even counter attacked curmudgeons who followed him in to class. Oh, wow! Now you're on the other side forgetting how recently it was you saying those very things to yours, truly. I didn't mind. This kind of 100% conversion is rare. I was proud of him.

So proud, that I got an idea from Kevin's success that I've continued to this day. Each class was given an official 'Loser of the Year'. I took the top person's weight loss and printed up a certificate proclaiming the achievement. It isn't the Oscars, but I feel it's no less important. I announced the winner of Kevin's class, with a year's total loss of 75#, KEVIN! He seemed genuinely touched. He was nonplussed. He came up, took the certificate (a mess, hand written in my sloppy penmanship. I've polished them up a lot since then), shared suggestions and sat back down.

After the meeting, he came up to me and thanked me with the most sincere tone I'd heard from him. He claimed that no one in his entire life had ever gone out of their way to acknowledge anything he'd accomplished in such a way. He didn't tear up, but he hesitated as he spoke. He said he'd never forget it. I didn't expect such a reaction. I was beyond proud of him.

After members make goal, some make the tragic mistake of thinking they're cured. They don't need to attend the meetings anymore. I cannot tell you how much I discourage this. No one gets a pass to permanent thin. If you stop doing the daily due diligent work, expect the pounds to return. I stress this point in meetings continuously. Some people, when they hear good advice, heed it. Others have to learn the hard way. I have had MANY members stop coming to classes, weighing in weekly and think they can do it on their own. Let me speak in provable facts here, not my own 2 cent opinion. I have had this proven to me over and over and over throughout the years. It's never over.

Kevin seemed to think he was an exception. A monthly weigh in at goal is the bare minimum required of members on the program to not pay. With his eye off the ball, the weight came back on. Kevin didn't want to pay. Kevin took the unwise approach of many before him by thinking he could recapture goal on his own. Evidently, my words about how this would happen echoed in his ears. BUT, he decided to prove me wrong. He was going to be the exception. No surprise, this never worked. Darn it, Kevin!

I was kept abreast of this by his thin family members who did not follow that strategy. They kept their weight off successfully for many years. I didn't ask about Kevin. It wasn't my business. I also knew if there was anything different to the story, they'd tell me. When I felt an adequate time period had passed, I tentatively broached it. The three of them huddled with me and said, with forlorn expressions, he was on the fast track to gaining all of it back. I was not surprised, but very sorry to hear this. I am never an "I told you so" who kicks anyone when they stumble. They said he was doggedly determined to prove me wrong. He was livid, furious that I was right. Sigh.

I'm not glad when I give advice that isn't taken and people fail. Never. I would welcome Kevin back with an open hand shake and no judgment if he walked back into my class tomorrow. Give the one who's watched 50,000 others try and see the credibility in what they're observed. I know what I know.

TIPS: See where credibility is. Kevin benefitted from family, me and the program. This was a powerful trifecta, indeed. Don't listen to people who are not practicing what they preach. Be objective about sources.

TRAPS: Pride goeth before a fall! Thinking you're cured is the quickest way to failure!

DON'T JUDGE A BOOK
BY ITS COVER:

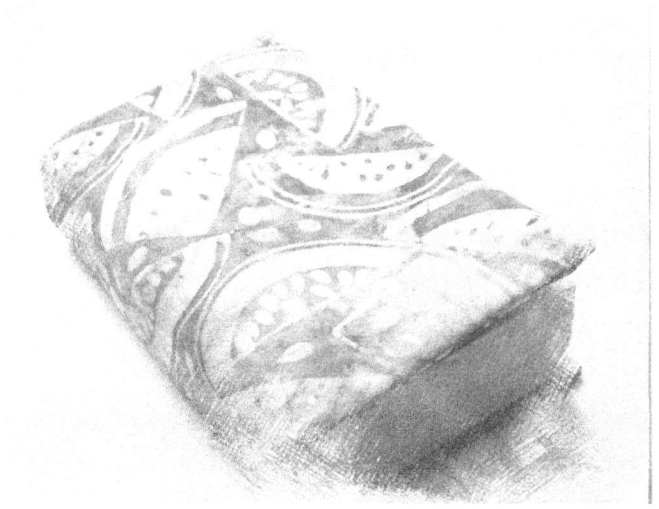

You can't judge a book by its cover. We've all heard this one and for good reason. Simply, it's true. I have been the recipient of negative prejudgments by more than a few people because when I teach my classes I'm usually dressed in very bright vibrant colors. They are my trademark. Hey, Minnie Pearl had her hat with the price tag and Johnny Cash had his 'all in black'. I spent many years only able to purchase clothes at the big men's store. Let me say, the choices were the only thing you'd call slim. Ugly colors and ugly clothes: black, brown, beige, slate gray, navy, icky off whites.

Nothing was pleasant to see. To add insult to injury, they were expensive. Not because of the need for more fabric, but because they know they've GOT you. If you're this size, big guy, you ain't goin' anywhere else. I'd leave feeling very down with $300 or so of stuff I didn't want, but needed. Then, a promise this was the last time I'd do this. I was going to lose weight, by golly and never go back. Well, tomorrow, maybe.

When I got slim, I decided that my sunny outlook should be matched by my clothes: the bolder and brighter the better. It was out of my hands how my members might react. Well, they loved it. It is the rare week I'm not in either basic but monochromatic bright or wacky patterns designed to make you smile: a costume, in a way. No need to shell out bucks to a shrink to see what made this turn around. Too many years in much too drab gear left me with the pendulum swinging the other, merrier way. May I never recover! Normal and I decided to see other people.

I like to think the best of everyone. It makes life more pleasant. Until you do or say something to make me see otherwise, I'll give you a chance. If you're friendly, we'll get along just fine no matter what your age, gender, weight, height, race, religion, political leaning, sexual orientation or any quirks of personality. In fact, I tend to like folks that have forged their own way by marching to their own drum deciding normal is overrated for them, too.

Some instances, it didn't happen. Everyone isn't on one beam. Given a chance, I like to win people over. Here are some examples:

SHANE:

A tall man of mid age with 60-70 extra pounds, a quiet type who sat in the back and didn't share much. Dressed in suits for work, I didn't get much of a feeling from him one way or the other. I always offer extra help to anyone who needs it. Shane seemed a very self-contained unit. He'd go and come back again with weight back on never opening up about his reasons for leaving, so I didn't ask. Shane wasn't hostile, but not friendly, either. We worked only on basics while he waited in line. The final time he'd rejoined, he got to goal. I gave him genuine hearty congratulations along with the class' loud applause. He asked to speak to me afterwards. Sure, Shane. He told me he wished to apologize for something. I had taken the class over from a teacher who'd been fired whom Shane was apparently very fond of. He said he'd hated me from the beginning, partially, because I wasn't 'her'. I knew this teacher's style and I am a completely different type than she was, so he'd found it too drastic. He felt everyone would also feel the same way and I'd be gone soon. So, he'd leave until I was dismissed and a more subtle, low key replacement would be in my place. He even called our local office from time to time asking if I was still there. The time and location were the only one he could attend, so he'd grudgingly rejoin with me, but not allow the program to work because he would not accept the message due to the messenger.

As he continued attending, he heard my stories, the heartbreaks I'd taken, the struggles with weight, the frustrations, the toll on my body... he also saw me interact with other members who were also trying to heal themselves. He said he was amazed at how much I connected with the class. Not only did no one else quit, but my attendance was higher than the previous leaders. I was running a better, more intimate class with more real program being practiced than he'd ever seen. He was impressed and ashamed of himself for thinking a man in head to toe orange was to be discounted on that basis alone. I thanked him for his candor. It took guts for him to admit this. I considered him a friend after that. He even smiled after that.

SANDRA:

Sandra joined with a friend for support. I've met 'I'm only here for them' people before. Often, it's a camouflage for their reluctance to admit they need help. I knew that was the case with Sandra. When I said my usual sunny hello, she backed off and looked at her friend like I was a Martian. While I admit it hurts to get this response, it's rare and comes with the territory of working with the public. I have had to acquire a poker face. Rolled eyes, snickers, exaggerated gawks were my usual greetings from Sandra. Her friend was quiet but seemed to relate to something in me and kept attending and losing weight. I never force anyone on the less boisterous side to speak in the meeting if that's not their thing. I work one on one with many members that may only open up in closer knit circles. Usually, she had her crutch Sandra with her. I learned to ignore her weekly routine of commenting on my attire, my toy clappers or my upbeat enthusiasm. Negativity and cynicism were Sandra's crutch. Time went on and her friend did well, indeed. Guess what, so did Sandra. She followed the program more out of social convenience due to her friend than anything else. No matter why, Sandra found herself happier and looking better and her quiet friend became more outgoing and had a change in personality for the better.

One night, Sandra raised her hand to speak. She said her work schedule was changing and she would not be able to attend my class anymore and so she had to say something. "I totally misjudged you. When I first met you, I couldn't stand you, anything about you. You were just too crazy. I was shocked my friend liked you and since I promised her I'd come along, that's the only reason I did. I asked her not to make me have to come and see this clown. But, wow, what you've been through. What you do for these people. What my friend has learned and the changes she's making in her life. (Sandra started crying) I really misjudged you. I have a tendency to judge a book by its cover and now I don't want to go to classes anymore if it isn't yours." I came in for a hug and Sandra didn't resist.

LORI'S MOM:

I met a chubby 12-year-old young lady named Lori who was joining with her mother. Lori was sweet faced and loved my colorful clothes. Her eating was only going to get better if her mother lead the way. She said she would and that was why she was joining, too. It was summer break and this was going to be their Saturday ritual. I was particularly funny that day. I thrive in front of a crowd. When the energy's right, I can open up their minds and hearts to receive essential information if they've laughed first. Lori always got a bit extra attention and blossomed as the weeks went by. Losing weight at this preadolescent stage is so crucial for a girl. She was going to endure enough changes that were out of her control. It was nice to see her work so hard at what she could control. As late August approached, Lori's mother asked to have a moment with me. No problem. I was sad to have to see them change days even though I knew from the start it would happen. Yes, that was one reason she was talking to me. The school year was a rearrangement of their time and they would have to seek another class. But, she said she felt the need to tell me that she'd been wrong about something. On the first day she'd joined, she didn't like me and was high tailing it out of there never to again be bothered with a flamboyant character like me. Way too over the top for her taste. If one's taste cannot include some over the top humor, I will never work for you. No worries, that's what other teachers are for. But, in the car Lori had said how much she liked me and how excited she was to start the program. She stared at Lori and I said, "you liked him?" "Yes, he's funny, mama! He made me feel like I can do this. He made me understand what I need to do and that I can't rely just on you, mom." I was amazed. Lori had never taken to anyone or anything to do with her extra weight before. So, I went for her sake back to your classes. Over the weeks, I got the serious messages you deliver. I heard the pain in your voice. I saw the joy in your face. I felt the concern for everyone in that room. My heart broke for both your struggles and for my own shame at my initial hasty judgment of you. I'm sorry." I miss Lori so.

I am sure there are many more out there, but these 3 individuals overcame their hesitation to trust someone who wasn't what they'd think was able to offer them anything of value based on nothing more than a first impression. All 3 got the program's message and emerged better for it. I won't change who I am to please all perspective joiners. I cannot reach everyone. No one can. But, I have learned to practice what I preach and am open to just about anyone I meet. An open book allows you to glimpse into others' worlds and enhance your own. Wisdom, grace and healing can happen anyplace.

TIPS: An open mind allows new information in - closed ones don't. You allow yourself to learn so much more when you don't seek knowledge solely from others like yourself.

TRAPS: If you truly don't like a teacher, it's likely they're not the only one. Find one who makes you feel open to learning. Quitting over an instructor accomplishes nothing useful for you.

RHONDA:

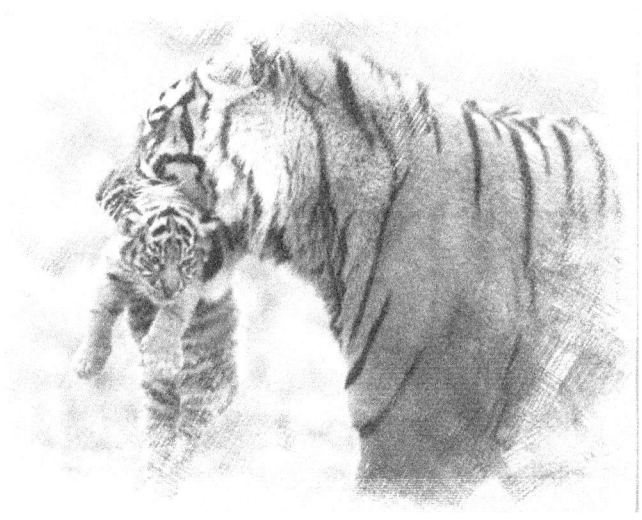

Rhonda: A dear lady. From the day she entered my meeting room and my life it was instant like and rapport. A petit thing, barely 5', but full of positive energy and with a willingness to alter her behaviors to allow the program to work its magic. In other words: an absolutely ideal joiner. With her happy attitude, you'd think Rhonda had it easy.

Then, I was privileged to meet her son. From the wheelchair I could not assess his condition entirely. I didn't ask because it was not my business, too. Also, that would be insensitive and I wanted very much to gain both of their trust. He seemed to have some physical deteriorations of the spine. A larger than average head, spoke with some difficulty, his arms and hands were not quite right. I still do not know his exact condition or how it came to be. Either from birth or an awful accident or a tragic malady, who knows? I really didn't care too much because, being Rhonda's son, he was also a delightful and pleasant young man. He'd obviously been loved and cared for and was flourishing as much as he could. When I see people in these circumstance, it reiterates how very blessed most of us are and how we blow minor inconveniences out of proportion. Yours truly is as guilty of this as anyone.

Rhonda took to the program well. Not coming in one time with a 'pity me and this terrible burden I have' excuse. How I'd love to clone her and show a streaming of it when weigh ins happen all over. It would knock the wind out of many members' excuse rolodex. We had a handicap capable scale, so I often took Rhonda and her son aside to weigh them in. It was usually good news for Rhonda. We'd pow-wow privately and I'd ask her if there were any special challenges she was facing and if I could at least offer guidance if it involved dining out or food. Sometimes all she wanted was a friendly ear. Her son was not too able to follow the program. Funny how human we all are: he sometimes fibbed to me or had other people get his snacks. Whoa! I'm kinda impressed! As a decades long sneaker of food myself, Rhonda's son was still finding ways to sidestep the program. Man, this is tough. I'd probably be like that, too!

Rhonda joined the gym, played tennis and had the natural love for activity so lacking in so many of the people I meet. As short as she was, the extra weight on her was not big in number, per se. But each pound shows so much more when you're under a certain height. She came in happier and more excited with her emergence from under the cocoon she'd been in. Often, she spoke up in meetings about how she was cooking new styles of food, making time to go to the gym, reading the material, not trying to cut corners since that'd never been successful in the past. I made sure to let the room know that if she was making time to do what needed to be done, why couldn't they? She put them to shame. But, perhaps they raised their own level of performance, too. I would have LOVED having Rhonda in my class.

It was more and more apparent that her son was opening up to me, too. Rhonda would glow with a mother's pride as he stuck out his hand, smiled and tried to express his thoughts to me week by week. Sometimes, people ignore handicapped people or treat them like they're babies - neither was true. Rhonda's son was a young man and a good one. He seemed like he didn't get enough plain old 'Hey, how are you, pal' type comments in his life. The healthier and happier Rhonda got, the surer I became that she would make goal and keep it off for good. Not a single doubt about it. Aerobics classes before or after weigh ins make Rhonda perpetually in gym clothes when I saw her. "I do own dresses", she'd say to me. "Smaller dresses, right?" I'd reply. "Man, you're good for my ego." I couldn't be more sincere, Rhonda. When the day happened that she made goal, I hugged her so hard I think I may have spun her around like a rag doll. Her advice wasn't profound for the room simply because it doesn't need to be. Eat sensibly, move more and mentally accept that it's a forever lifestyle change and PRESTO, you're thin. Rhonda got a standing ovation.

I saw Rhonda regularly as she lit up the place any morning she was there. Then, I didn't see her for a while. She seemed less happy when she returned. I had to ask her, in private, if everything was alright. Code, I suppose, for if her son was alright. She only said, she'd been in a very dark place and it'd been very tough and she'd put on a few pounds and was embarrassed to come back to my class. But, she needed to very badly.

I cannot express how unnecessary it is for members to avoid their teacher if they've slipped up, gained back weight or feel like they'll be criticized. I have met other teacher's members avoiding them, too. Nothing could be further from the truth, I can speak for any teacher I've come across, just come back. You'll get a judgement-free hug and welcome back. This unhappy Rhonda didn't suit her well.

It was apparent when she brought her son the next week that he'd gained weight considerably. Well, that's part of it. He was not willing or able to do the program. I'm leaning more towards willing, since I do believe he was perfectly capable mentally if he took more interest and initiative. Sigh.

When she brought him back to rejoin, he didn't have his regular chair with him. How were we to weigh him, then? Rhonda had been through this whole routine. We knew what she weighed - check. This warrior mother picked this heavy person up with her arms and strong back out of his chair with no help from him - truly, he was just 'weight' she was lifting - I got the number. She put him back in his chair, I subtracted her weight and we knew what he now weighed. I was so stunned, saddened, impressed and surprised by what I'd seen that words didn't come, at first. When they did, I was mad at the politically correct / human resources side to what did - 'Rhonda, from a legal stance, I can't help you pick your son up.' 'I know. I've had to do this many times.'

After a little while, they stopped coming again. I wrote a couple of postcards beseeching Rhonda to return. As of 5 months since my last one, she has not. I believe I will see her again. She's too mighty and driven to live under too much weight. While my pleas have so far been unanswered, my prayers are with her and my admiration, too. We will meet again.

TIPS: Never prejudge thin people in a weight loss room. You never know what struggles they're possibly facing. Also, do you need all ducks in a row to succeed, NO! Be flexible. The only sure thing is change. Be ready and have a plan B. You'll likely need it.

TRAPS: Avoiding program until you lose weight is like not going to a doctor until a wound heals on its own or you stitch it yourself. It just doesn't make good sense. Just come back.

FELICIA:

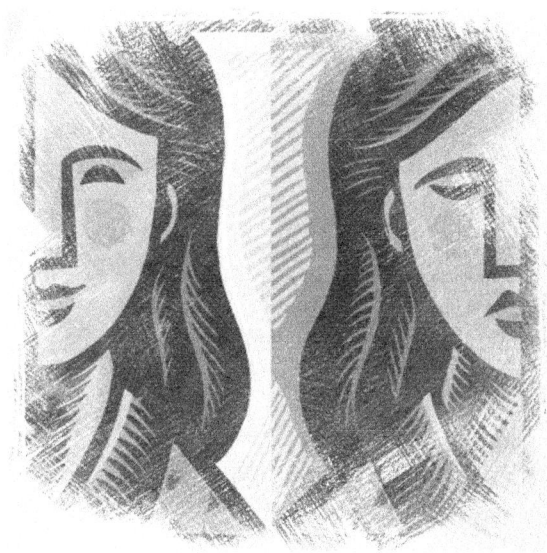

When I joined the program my umpty-umph and final time, it was different from the start. I wanted to lose the weight. I was never willing to do what needed to be done. I could FEEL the happy surrender in my blood as I drove there. Of course, I still ate 2 Hostess fruit pies on my way to the first meeting. Some things don't change. For full details about my epiphany, see my chapter.

I teacher shopped briefly. I did not like my first one. She was very popular. Nevertheless, I just didn't cotton to her style. While it was the most convenient time and location, I had to switch until I found the right person. This lead me to a teacher that I dug from the first time we met. I obediently followed her guidance and the weight came off. I will be grateful to her forever.

Well, amongst the things she did was put an employment application in my hand before I was even at my goal weight. I was close and she said I was going to be a teacher. "Oh, I am?" Well, I did whatever she said and it was working out tremendously, so this was no exception. My open interview with other prospective teachers was daunting. This was an entirely different type of endeavor than I'd been involved with. Also, the other man there was a school teacher. I thought I was cooked. Coming here was a waste of time. Little did I know, this was not a liability. My training director told me later school teachers can be too agenda driven, given to lecturing instead of interacting, have an 'I know this and you don't' mind set and are also often, well, dull. OK, then.

When you're selected to become a new teacher you're assigned to an established one for a 4 week mentoring period. This is where I met Felicia: my mentor, my vessel into a profession that would turn my life upside down both job wise and personally.

Felicia was a New Yorker. How can I put this - she was what some people would call a stereotypical New Yorker? Weather that's a good or bad thing is up to you. What I mean is she was loud, opinionated, edgy, sarcastic, quick witted, cynical and funny as heck! But she was not for the sensitive, easily offended or those who simply cannot grasp satire in thought or speaking. I don't know if she was Italian or Jewish, but she was one of those 2 and I felt it too personal to ask.

Felicia had a following that hung onto her every word. She could have been a stand-up comedian. Well, she really WAS a stand-up comedian. She just worked the program centers instead of night-clubs. It wasn't all fun and frivolity in her classes. No. No. She'd lost over 1OO# which at a petite 5'2" was a transformation that would impress anyone! She'd left an unfulfilling job she'd stayed at far too long due to a lack of confidence from being obese, too. Wow, she was a LOT like me! Also, she was gracious enough to share her spotlight with me. Not all teachers like doing this, I'd later discover.

So, I'm introduced to a chagrined group that did NOT come here to meet me. I was glad then that I have a weight loss that is large. Fair or not, it's gotten me some open minded reactions from new members that smaller weight losses do not. I feel genuinely sorry for leaders that have to face resistance from obese members who look at their 25 or less pound loss with less than co-operative minds simply because they were smart enough to not get morbidly obese in the first place.

First session, I am introduced, give a brief self-disclosure and observe. When Felicia took the meeting back, she went into a shtick of Baba Wawa interviewing Katherine Hepburn. Baba Wawa was Gilda Radner's (of the original 'Saturday Night Live' cast) funny rendition of Barbara Walters. Famously, she exaggerated Ms. Walters' slight lisp to hilarious effect. WHY was Felicia having the character talking to Katherine Hepburn? You got me? The room seemed confused as the unfunny story was playing out. It was a rare misfire from Felicia.

What Felicia didn't know was that I do some impressions. A mimic from childhood, I grasp onto many dialects and accents somewhat well: Katherine Hepburn, included. Her shaky, low, vibrating articulate, heavily mannered way of speaking —I can do it. So, the moment was there. But, don't forget, I didn't know Felicia well enough to know how she'd react to my interrupting her class. It was now or never.

I cleared my throat and said in a darn good Kate H.: "Personally, Barbara, I don't know what you're getting at." The class ROARED with laughter. The timing was perfection. Comics will always say that timing will make or break any set up. The funniest sketch in the world can tank with poor timing or delivery. She walked behind the easel, acknowledging her moment being taken from her. What a sport! I apologized for taking this chance later on, but she simply wouldn't have it. "Look. I'm funny. I know I'm funny and you completely took that moment away from me and made it yours. Not an easy thing to do." Whew, I was worried. She told me she was never worried about my ability to be a good teacher after that.

Fine tuning was all I required. Some things only experience will give you. Training can only go so far. Amongst my areas I would need the most help was in the joiners' orientation. That was an entirely new vista for me. The meeting has as much to do with interaction, reading people's faces, hearts, words, involving others to create a bonded and safe environment that's conducive to learning. The orientation is more basic info. My first one didn't go well. I was green and my maiden voyage tanked. When we spoke afterwards, Felicia let me know this. I knew it, too. She said my first big mistake was asking the joiner what the impetus was that got them to join: a good ice breaker. No one joins the program out of the clear blue. Something happened. We all know this. No. Her objection was the word 'impetus'. I tried to tell her it meant the final occurrence that got them to .... "I KNOW what it means." Felicia cut me off. "Look, you haven't worked with the public in a long time. I have. The word's too big. You say 'What made you join? Or something simple like that. There are some stupid f in' people out there. You're about to meet a lot of them." This is typical Felicia style and she wasn't wrong. Blunt speaking is something I take to well. It helped. I never used 'impetus' again. There are some stupid people out there. But, they deserve the benefits that the program can offer. So, if I need to drop my vocabulary back to 6th grade to reach more people, I'll do it. I'm no snob.

Sadly, Felicia herself regained her weight. Teachers have to be at goal. Whatever personal insecurities she was battling got the better of her. She was SO popular, the rules were bent for her and she was teaching classes while she was gaining. She would discuss it openly with her members. I'm sure most forgave her, but newcomers would look at her and say, "THAT'S the teacher? She's heavier than I am!" It couldn't go on. Felicia was let go after a considerable amount of time was given to her to re lose her weight with the offer of returning if she ever did. She never got thin again from what I hear. I would LOVE to pay it forward and have her join my class and let me help her. Open invitation, girl. I'm waiting. Smiling.

TIPS: Take risks. If you're blessed to know you're dying (I, personally, want to know) a common regret people say they have is they wish they'd taken more risks. Felicia took risks. I did, too. Both of us altered our lives for the better for it.

TRAPS: Don't give of yourself until there's nothing left for you. Noble doesn't mean masochist. As far as I'd observed, this got the better of Felicia.

HEATHER AND DON:

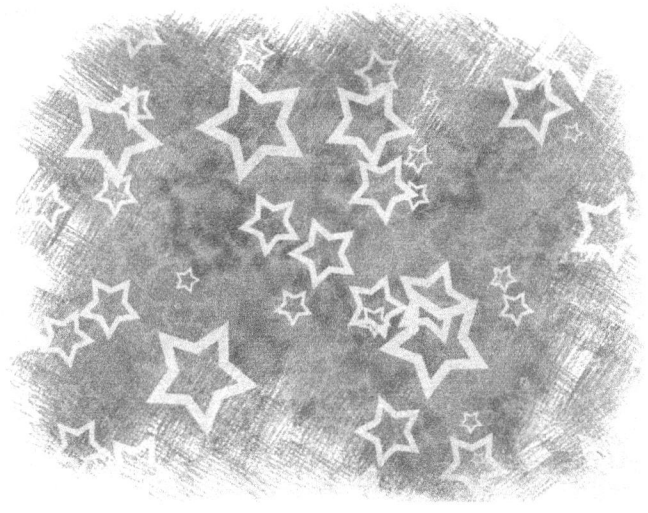

Heather joined the program with her husband Don. A petite silver haired lady: well dressed, well-spoken and obviously intelligent. Like people her size, the extra 30# on Heather was enough to keep her from living the life she wanted to, slow her down and affect her morale. Taking the bull by the horns, she simply would not have it. Joining with her husband seemed like the ideal arrangement. Don was a sweet tempered man with nearly 100 extra pounds. However, his enthusiasm seemed mediocre. I sensed that the relationship between them was long ago set regarding food, eating and his health. It went this way: he didn't do anything about any of it. Heather cooked, cleaned, made any adjustments for various diets they'd take on and push for doctor's appointments against a very resistant spouse.

I turned out to be absolutely right about this. Heather would come to class, ask questions, write down notes and seemed open to the direction of the topics, no matter where they went. My faith in her was justified. The weight came off and Heather became another triumph against the too often accepted excuses that a woman over a certain age cannot get thin. The blossoming of her world was reflected in the colorful sunny dresses she'd come in each week. Practically beaming with happiness as I commented on the particular patterns and the sizes - Heather was going to get the rewards for the change in lifestyle she was undertaking. I was so very happy for her.

Goal was Heather's soon after and I knew she'd be successful in maintaining afterwards. She'd been ready - all in from the start. When someone joins in this state, my job is much simpler. All credit goes to the member and the program —I only facilitate the journey. In the years since then, Heather has kept it off and made it look easy. My OWN maintenance isn't this smooth. I can only hope to have Heather's will. Age hasn't slowed her down or affected her good mood or her 'every week is May Day' style of dressing. She's adapted to the programs tweaking and changes without balking or clinging to the past because she trusts the program. Again, a rare and delightful open mindedness that I suggest anyone who wants to remain slim forever adopt. Heather is amazing!

Now, if that were all of it, it would be like a fairy tale that did, indeed, come true. Real life is where Heather lived and did her work. Don was the opposite of Heather. I hear opposites attract. Where Heather was pleasant, Don seemed glum. She met your eyes and Don looked down. Her hugs and handshakes were firm and unforced. Don gave me the 'dead fish' handshake that I find extremely off putting - particularly in men. She asked questions, he seemed like he wanted to be anywhere but where he was. On the few times I made the miscalculation of trying to gently engage Don, I got mumbled and barely intelligible replies that trapesed off into the mist. Don never got very far and Heather showed her overreaching by asking questions that pertained to him on his behalf. This never works. All the good intentions in the world always backfire when one spouse tries to do all the leg work for the other. If they are not actively involved in their own recovery, it's a cause that's lost.

This is common enough that it still wouldn't have been enough to include this couple. No, it came from what was revealed slowly as Don would join up with Heather over and over through the years. Always welcomed back with a smile, he'd say something about how this time he was ready to take this seriously due to some malady that was bothering him. Fine, I was a multi-joiner, too. I understand that.

Meanwhile, a pattern was repeated of Heather asking all the questions while Don passively sat there. I'd try to focus on him and ask him about the literature in an effort to motivate him to become at least a co participant in his own recovery. He suffered from depression. I found out. What was he depressed over? I asked. "Just depression", was his answer. I have met so many people like this that somehow manage to marry their opposite. I wonder if the women think that they'll change them. If they feel so sorry for them and it gets mixed with other feelings, they mistake for love. I don't know the inner facets of Don and Heather's marriage and it's not my business. Only in the ways it was blocking any attempts for Don to succeed did I care.

Heather was succeeding and made it look easy, as I'd said. Turns out, her home environment was anything but easy. She was keeping up her food discipline while Don kept all manner of fattening foods around them. He was as inconsiderate of her efforts as possible. If she was going to be thin, it was to be tested while she bought, cooked and lived with all the snacks Don was unwilling to live without. Heather has to take part of the blame for this. It was her own choice to accept this and put herself in this toughest as possible situation. However, Don was oblivious to what a position he was putting his wife in for keeping the family peace. Not everyone shares their struggles and stresses with the world. Heather was such a case. Some people wear their troubles on their sleeve and talk of them constantly. Heather soldiered on privately. Now I saw how much the classes were her lifeline. I know I have a very important job. Some people have no other support system but the classes. I take that seriously. If they're to get any encouragement, education, examples, cooking advice, guidance, feedback or sanity - It's in the classes.

When Don rejoined at about the 12-year mark of my first meeting them, he said the same things he'd said before. I had a heart to heart conversation with him and Heather that this needed to be his journey or there was no point in him rejoining. He bad to be the #1 person involved and Heather must not rush in and take the leg work away from him. Don was not a child. It seemed that when the enabling stopped, Don took to his role as pilot. I was encouraged by this new behavior following the too many times said words. The magic of action was happening. This was a most unexpected, but gloriously good sign.

Don is 60+# down and seems to have the Heather circa 2006 fire in him. He's losing, speaks up, asks his own questions, reads his own leaflets and his smile is genuine, he looks me in the eye, gives off a relaxed demeanor and I couldn't be prouder. I truly had written Don off. I am GLAD to say I was wrong.

Most touching of all, when Don hit 50#, we gave him his due applause and a token to note the achievement. Don spoke with cracks on the verge of tears when he shared how he was proud of what he was doing, but he now saw the strain he'd put on his wife. He was losing, but living in a 100% supportive environment entirely in sync with the program. He had been a constant adversary in Heather's way and now he recognized it. He said she was so strong, so amazing, so patient, he could never, ever had been able to do this if the person he lived with was behaving as he'd done. He was very contrite. Heather deserved to hear this. I didn't even say the standard, 'Oh, that's alright' to let him off the hook for this. It hadn't been alright. It had been cruel - whether it was intentional or not. Now, Don saw this and owed Heather the apology. With that now said, I see Don in a new light. He is discovering what he's capable of and weighs less than he's weighed in over 40 years. Another senior superstar! Now, THAT's the fairy tale ending. May they live happily, thin-ly ever after.

TIPS: Marry Heather! She may not have shown it, but she had a tough home environment to face. She needed the classes, took notes, asked questions, followed up on assignments. If you have a lifeline, use it well.

TRAPS: Letting someone else do your work doesn't pay off. You're left unskilled, unable to walk alone and are as vulnerable as a house of cards. Crawl, walk - then, run. You are wise to ask for help, but avoid pawning off your whole endeavor.

NICK:

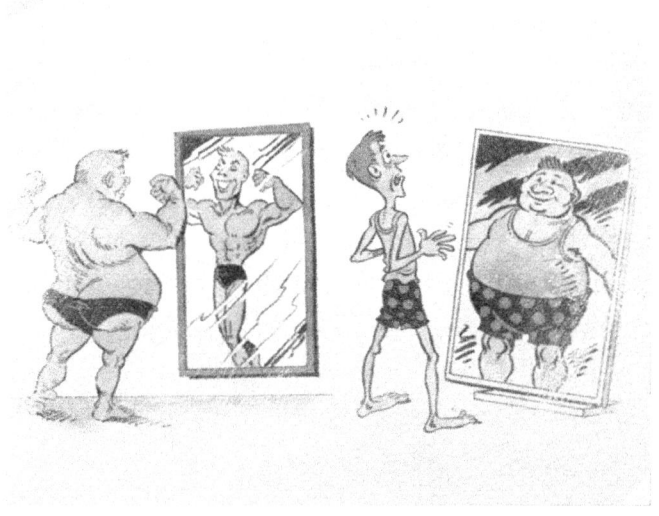

"I'm in perfect health. I've been to a doctor and he told me. So, don't give me any s**t about it, there's nothing wrong." How I wish I could take you all with me back to this day when this line was flung at me like a load of, well, what he'd said. Nick was 440+# and evidently, in fine shape. It remains one of my ultimate unforgettable statements I've ever heard. My receptionist and I still talk about it to this day.

Looking far braver than I felt, I replied, 'Then why are you here?' Wow, I couldn't believe I'd looked big Nick right in his biker face and met his line in the sand with mine. He was struck silent and I survived. Whew! Maybe his wife that had joined with him was why? It was her idea, it turned out. Didn't see that corning! I wanted to add,

'Oh, and, by the way, the doctor that told that line to you is a 100% certified quack. Don't ever see him again.' But, I thought the better of it and stilled my tongue.

There was so much wrong with Nick that it overwhelmed me to think about where to begin. The basics seemed the only reasonable way. My greatest counter attack to his great wall of denial came when I told him (and showed him photo evidence) that I'd been over 400#. THAT rocked him a bit. I SAW it in his eyes. Ah, the eyes never lie. He was clearly not expecting this. I don't know what went through his mind, but he was assured by me that I knew how he felt, had endured it for years, knew likely pretty close to how much he was eating and what a walking time bomb of maladies he was. He couldn't get away with any crap with me. I wasn't going to let him. I KNEW the drill. He could accept it and we'd move forward or stick his head back in the sand. He stayed. Oh, he sneered and grimaced when I made statements like 'you cannot find love in your fridge' and 'the rest of this day is not a free day'. I thought he'd punch me. Lucky for me, he just shook his head. But, he kept corning back.

Nick was very intimidating. A biker, multiple tattoos, engineer boots, chain wallet, doo rag wrapped around a shaved bald head, Van Dyked around the mouth. He looked like a psychotic Burl Ives. Other members sat as far away from him as possible. It was sometimes embarrassing. He and his wife would be in a section alone while 20 members were on the other side. He was accustomed to being able to throw his weight around literally and figuratively and quite unused to being challenged. I know I won his respect by letting him know I wasn't going to take any nonsense from him (in a non-confronta-tional way, of course, not in a smoke filled bar over a pool game). He had an 8-year-old son that I thought must be terrified beyond belief of him. He was well mannered and behaved, to my surprise. See, you never know.

Nick's wife seemed to be some warped version of June Cleaver. She looked like she should be Nick's lady. Her get-up being suitably compatible to his, she was no stranger to the back of a few motorcycles. But, she spoke sweetly and had that 'mother' tone to her. I began to see there was soil that could be cultivated here. They would take care of it and the harvest could begin. The program opened up Nick to a vista of products that he'd been unaware of. No surprise, his primary foods were wings, beer, bread, onion rings, potato skins... typical bar food for someone that probably had spent most of his life in 'em. Nick looked for all kinds of reduced calorie treats to gnaw on. Weekly,

I was more and more happily surprised by his gushing over what new thing he'd found. Most of the time, I was aware of it already, but I would never have cut him off. He was getting such a kick out of every new cookie, hot dog, chip, cake, bean dip, cracker, cereal, wheat bread, margarine, pretzel, grilled chicken on sticks, pudding, hamburgers unadorned with so much goo they were slipping out .... I would just beam with pride in Nick. Never judge a book by its cover, I always say. So, I am glad to live it regarding others, too.

No surprise, at Nick's size, the weight came off very quickly. The first hundred pounds was gone in less than 6 months. It is a considerable feat - but, premature for too much celebrating. After all, going from 443 to 340 isn't even 1/2 way. I was worried when the inevitable would happen. My concern was how Nick would respond when the guaranteed losses slowed down. There was a lot of extra fat on his body that had been there a long time and it would fight him. Hard lard, I call it. Nick was a fighter, I know. But, I would be his corner man and make sure that, at least, he wouldn't be sucker punched by it. He'd get notice.

Meanwhile, Nick's spark was contagious and he went from someone that was avoided and hostile to one of the most involved members in the room: a dream student, really. I had to hold onto the podium when a newbie said something about how they were unable to lose weight for same oft used excuse and Nick spoke up that that was just an excuse and he'd have to be 'real' and 'get with the program'. THIS from a guy who'd stubbornly insisted he was 440 pounds of good health. Some things are best forgotten.

Nick's wife lost a lot of weight, too. The teamwork they had was a model for couples. I have had many couples join together and as often as not when one of them does better than the other or there is an imbalance in the reasons they're there or motivations are not on the same level - well, it doesn't work well. Nick and his lady were in sync with dining out, food shopping, researching, not buying foods or sodas for the house that would tempt them. He seemed happy and proud of her when she hit 50# off. She seemed happy and proud of him at 100#. What a pair. As clothes needed replaced, they went to the store with mutual bliss at the sizes dropping. I know what it felt like to see the XXXL become a XXL. Nick's discovery of his own body in a new light was something I understood and rejoiced for him.

A new job required a move to another class in another part of town and a switch to a center I didn't teach at. I have to tell you I was very sad to see them go. Reluctant to let any other leader take the reins from me. Get their hands on 'em. Protective of Nick because he was a unique case and special handling was needed. Perhaps, too proudly, but I felt I was the best leader for him. But, making a living pulls all of us in directions we must accept. I found out who their new teacher would be and she's great. I called her beforehand to let her know what to expect and a bit of their back story. She told me how he took over meetings with 'my old teacher said this' and 'my old teacher said that' and she also had a kind yet firm way with teddy bears like Nick. I know Nick and his wife are thin people under construction. They'll be fine.

TIPS: Overweight people often have selective vision and hearing. They see what they want to see and hear what they want to hear. Healthy choices were always there. They were to the left, to the right, above or below the junk you bought that made you overweight. You just didn't see them until your eyes were opened.

TRAPS: Denial. If thinking you're healthy at 400+# doesn't speak for itself, nothing can.

VINCE:

When I met Vince, it was not a pleasant experience. His 400+# body wasn't the reason. His unkempt appearance was everything people with negative stereotypes about the obese claim they all have. His hair was flat and greasy. His clothes were wrinkled, old and obviously of no concern to him. Worst of all was his smell. It greeted you long before you could shake his hand. I know the smell. How can I best describe it —I call it 'fat man smell'.

Having been over 400# myself, I spent much effort ensuring that I did not have it. When your folds of fat are as plentiful and large as

Vince's, sweating is inevitable. If it doesn't get proper attention, the sweat simply has nowhere to go.

This accumulates and causes the unpleasant scent. It's not that part that's off putting to me. It's that it's fixable and he chose not to. In my own daily routine was powder and Shower to Shower underneath all my fat flaps: under my arms, under my 'man breasts' (larger than most women I've met) and under my gargantuan stomach. In the shower, I'd literally lift them up with one hand and soap and rinse them with the other to make sure they were as clean as possible. The powder routine was the needed follow up so that during the days of Las Vegas summer heat, I would avoid smelling like Vince.

Why do some obese and overweight people ignore themselves on such a basic level? I'm not even saying presenting themselves in a fashionable way. I'm talking basic hygiene. It's inexcusable to me. Frankly, the more overweight you are, the MORE you need to pay attention to these details, not less. Have all the ones whom I've seen in public that followed Vince's way just stopped caring, thus, stopped trying? "What's the point? I'm already so far gone." It's some people's rationale, I suppose. I saw it the opposite way. I am glad to say that no matter how huge I got, I was always clean, washed, showered, shaved, in pressed clothes, my hair neatly combed and sprayed ....as presentable as possible.

The kicker for Vince was that when he spoke, it was clear that he was a very intelligent man: a computer whiz, of all things. Computers and technology are both things I'm woefully behind in. My knowledge of these areas is likely surpassed by the average eight year old. But I digress. Vince was working simultaneously on programs for his own start-up company and working various jobs for others. Hmmm.

OK. When I told him that I'd been his size, that I'd experienced his level of struggle and I knew the pain and limitations he was living with - I hoped it'd open up his eyes, mind and heart to the possibility that he, too, could accomplish his weight loss goals. What were the odds that he'd walk into a center and find a male teacher (most are female) who'd been in such a similar situation? <u>This could have worked out so well!</u>

Alas, that was not the case. Vince was one excuse after another. Unsuccessful launches were followed by mumbled reasons why he was just too busy to concentrate on the program this week and next week might be different. I'd listen - never critical or suggesting he was being judged - and ask him basic questions that would get replies I knew were just not true. Yes, he did the program right. Why didn't he lose? This week, his computer company had a major crash, so .... that meant he had to go to whatever fast food place he was at .... on and on this went.

I know in cases of the obese, weight losses and regains happen in bigger numbers than those with less weight to lose. In a period of five to six months, Vince not only didn't lose any weight, he weighed more than when he started. He skipped classes. Unbeknownst to him, a church acquaintance of his worked with me and reported seeing him out socially from time to time. Always eating, doing nothing to help himself. This knowledge only further contributed to my difficulty reaching him since I KNEW he was lying to me; it was an insult to be lied to so regularly.

I'm in class to help people. Food is an insidious problem. There is much insincerity involved. I'm lied to on a constant basis. I, myself, was no stranger to that game. As if lying to your weight loss counselor is going to matter when you step on the scale. 'Your body doesn't play that game. "If you didn't see me eat it, I didn't eat it." No one wins that one. I wonder how many times a weight loss counselor rolled their eyes at me as I told juicy non truths about what I did or didn't do that week. Mamma Mia!

BUT, this makes me a strong teacher. You can't con me too much. A reformed con artist knows how to read between the lines very well. I am the one who has to call them on it, always emphasizing that I've been there and with offers of potential ways to improve. Not just being berated. I know that doesn't work. But I will tell people the truth without worrying about if it's what they want to hear. That's my job. Not all people appreciate this, believe me.

In that vein, Vince would have meandered through the ongoing months for who knows how long. But, I was forced to address his unpleasant body odors. Others would not sit within as many seats of him as possible. They'd take folding chairs and move them to avoid him. Crowded lines always seemed to have space in front of or behind Vince. It was a business. It was a problem and I knew it had to be dealt with. After conferring with my boss, I took him aside and said some members had spoken to me about his body odor and it would have to be improved for him to continue. He didn't defend it or argue. He said he'd put some attention into it and simply sat down. Was this the first time he'd heard this? Probably not. With no progress and his evidently endless work his computer program business was taking, Vince just fell out of the program. It wasn't a surprise. If he'd have succeeded, that would have surprised me. But I do know that I went out of my way to help him for months. But he remained unreceptive, to my dismay.

Fast forward to me in a supermarket and he and his wife (yes, he was married - which somehow surprised me) turn one corner and I, the other. We say hello. I asked about his work. His wife said he'd mentioned me after weigh in's. I wanted to ask what he said, but decided I didn't really want to know. He was going to come back some time. I said, I hope so and the door was always open. I reminded him I'd been a multiple joiner, too, and that was that. Never saw him again.

If you recall, I said he had a fellow church parishioner I worked with. A couple of years later, he asked if I remembered Vince? Sure, I said. "His funeral's Monday". Damn it! Damn it! This didn't have to happen. This obviously intelligent man was dead at 40 something. One emotion I could not say I felt was surprise. You can only tempt fate & abuse the body for so long: a tragic ending.

I know if I had not taken myself in hand, only one of two things would have been my future. Take the passing years and the weight gain train of disaster I was riding multiplied = I would be one of those shut in cases. 800#, 900# - they don't even look like human beings anymore. Can't move, wipe themselves.... but, they sure still manage to eat. OR, I'd be dead. The heart is only a muscle. It can't be taxed to such a level forever. I know there wasn't an option three. Of the two, if I were allowed to choose, I'd choose dead. Nothing tastes good enough for you to depart this world a decade too soon… nothing.

TIPS: No size is beyond fixing. No matter what your current size, take heart, take courage and take the first step. It's fixable. It's still not too late.

TRAPS: Sadly, one day it IS too late: your last day on Earth. You cannot ignore morbid obesity. It won't go away or even remain status quo. Your body will rebel and you may not survive the rebellion.

TAMMY, FROM A TINY NEVADA TOWN:

In a busy church room, in a chaotic atmosphere, with a lot of noise and people to deal with — I stopped at the sight of Tammy, from a small Nevada town as she walked in the door to join. Well, walked is not quite the right word. Hobbled, maybe? How do I describe her? I'd better be objective, at first. She was hunched over on a walker going about ¼ a mile per hour. Every move seemed to cause her pain. Her hair looked like a gray bird's nest. It was dirty, un- brushed and had too many home remedies of color attempts. Her muumuu was gigantic and formless. No doubt in an effort to conceal the

120+# of extra weight on her 5'3" or so frame. Her face was weather beaten and red from living in the middle of the desert. Her breath, when she spoke, stunk and was off putting. This is what I saw.

Who I met touched my heart. She could barely say more than a sentence without needing to stop from shortness of breath. Indeed, she lived in a small remote little town in isolation. All she did was eat junk and watch TV. Grown kids were gone and on their own. She did not work, maybe never had. I didn't ask. She'd been scared by a visit to a doctor and that's what brought her to the program. I didn't need details about her state of health yet. Just by looking at her and hearing her I knew she was a laundry list of maladies. Take one thing at a time. She'd walked in the door. It was her sweetness that I saw underneath the desperation that melted my heart. I wanted to help her.

Her husband: missing some teeth, with a prospector's hat, grungy boots and dungarees. He spoke like he was auditioning for 'Return to the Ponderosa'. What a pair they were. They seemed like characters from a corny old Western movie. Tammy, from a tiny Nevada town was 'allowed' to come here and do this because the doc said she had to. I gulped down my desire to give a sarcastic reply. Women who are under a man's thumb bring out a protective streak in me. But, I certainly didn't want to offend. Also, I thought, somewhat grandly, perhaps, that if I didn't help her — she'd just give up.

I allowed Tammy, from a tiny Nevada town to bypass the long line since standing for long periods of time was so difficult. She appreciated it. To my delight, the sweet nature I saw in her was genuine and we struck up as much of a friendship as a weight loss teacher / student relationship. Pain was her initial motivation. It's a great one, very effective, too. We went week by week and she took notes (a habit

I love) and made her husband stop at the grocery store on their way back to get what they needed after class. She was obviously someone who'd been in the background most of her life, no one paying too much attention to her. Tammy, from a tiny Nevada town blossomed when someone asked her questions, heard her reply, offered guidance and encouraged her to participate in conversations. Like a dying flower that was given water, sunshine and fertile soil just in the nick of time, Tammy, from a tiny Nevada town sprung to life!

Her fondness for cooking had fallen to the wayside as frozen junk had become the primary food supply for her. Nothing nutritious seemed to enter her mouth. She bought cookbooks and studied them. Next week, we'd all hear her delightful excitement as she got surprisingly good results from lighter recipes. Also, her husband was glad to have fresh home cooked meals, too. Vitality became her new medicine. Weekly, she improved and I always congratulated her on her awakened self- worth. She bought new clothes. I was so happy. She came in with make up on. I was smiling ear to ear. She joined a ladies' gym and did her best and moved more. I was her #1 admirer. When she came in having a new hairdo from the beauty parlor, I said, 'Look at you, glamour girl!' She was beaming with pride. She found a local discount place that also took to her new style. She was unstoppable.

About the time Tammy, from a tiny Nevada town was closing in on 100# off, she bested all her previous morphing. She walked in unassisted. I mean walked in. She'd already graduated from a walker to a cane that she leaned on more than relied on. She stood in the door, with erect posture and looked at me. I came over and hugged her (probably too hard!) unconcerned with anyone else there for at least a minute. She cried and thanked me. She'd done it for herself. But, I was honored and glad to have played a part in the journey. She shared that she was off her entire load of meds she was on. Her doctor was astounded at her. Tammy, from a tiny Nevada town saved her life. Nothing less.

Then one night, she asked to speak to me alone. She told me that when she joined, she'd been living in such isolation and was so miserable she'd been suicidal. Her husband liked the situation, but Tammy, from a tiny Nevada town curled up and nearly died in their hot, lonely trailer in the middle of nowhere she'd been dragged to. Thinking she would never be able to alter her destiny, she ate with abandon. The big secret was that her husband knew she wanted to leave and move back to civilization. She had him promise if she lost all her weight, he'd agree. Well like someone saying they'll quit smoking on a bet they think they'll never lose, here Tammy, from a tiny Nevada town was - doing what she said she'd do. Now, he was beginning to see that she expected him to make good on his part of the bargain. She was too happy and too full of life to stay stuck in the sticks. Happily, he did honor his word to his wife.

Only, this meant I had to say 'goodbye'. How could I? She was 120# lighter, but still about 40 or so more pounds to goal. She was moving far away and had no ties to where she was, so it was unlikely we'd meet again. This was before Facebook, Linked in and such. I had to trust her that she'd join another program center and finish the journey. She was worried she'd not like it with a different leader. NO, I couldn't let her foster even the slightest hesitation about continuing due to looking backwards on account of me. I loved Tammy, from a tiny Nevada town. But, she needed to lock arms in her new town.

We hugged, she cried, I kept my lumpy throat at bay while I wished her well, made her promise over and over that she was going to keep losing weight. I have not seen too many more shining examples of someone turning their life around to that degree in all my years of weight loss counseling. Tammy, from a tiny Nevada town, I love you.

TIPS: Isolation is damaging to many folks. Now, you can be much more connected for informational purposes to the world. It's much better than it was. Low self-esteem opens doors to many unhappy places. Tammy, from a tiny Nevada town nearly let it consume her. But, she went where she had to go, buy what she needed to have and overcame!

TRAPS: If your husband wants to move you to the middle of nowhere to live in a trailer with little to no contact with the outside world, unless this is a mutual desire, say, "NO"!

PAULA:

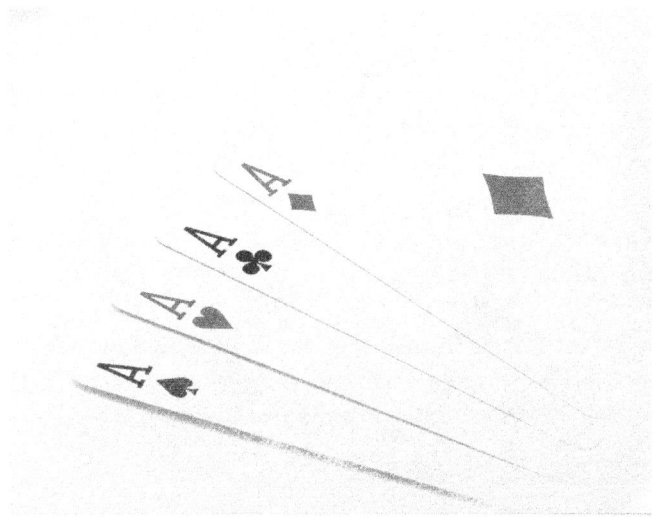

Paula is the kind of person others are happy to see. Blond, fare skinned, pretty, unassuming, easy to smile and generous with her time, love and talents...seems the ideal wife, mother, friend and, as it turned out, student of mine.

Being overweight brought an unnatural glumness to Paula. I do not know if her positivity came from her upbringing or if it was inert in her. I do find nature over nurture observations very interesting. Being overweight was slowing her down and bringing her confidence down with it. Also raising children with the excess baggage was clouding

Paula's sunshine. Life takes patience, family takes more of it; children take infinite patience and energy. Paula had had enough.

Not too overweight, but enough that her quality of life was impacted. That is the accurate diagnosis for Paula. 35— 40# off and she'd be beautiful, youthful looking and able to tackle life's challenges with ease and invite much more joy into it. Dieting had not worked for her. She was stuck. But Paula found inspiration in the program and I became quite fond of her. She brought her kids to see me and they were charming and well mannered. I do suspect she was raised by quality parents. The apple didn't fall far from the tree.

Paula became immersed in the program. Offering thoughtful comments and rejoicing in each victory. Saying 'no, thank you' to tempting foods. Trying to cope with life's daily stresses and not looking for relief via eating. Having her husband's support was an asset I was glad she had. It makes a HUGE difference when the people you live with are on the same page and allow the necessary environmental changes to ease the way.

I heard Paula talk of exercising. I heard her talk of showing her children how to use the tools she used. I could see that my overweight experiences as a kid touched her. I know she did not want her own children to suffer. It was in her hands to lead the way by practicing what she would preach. Deemphasizing food, cooking and being the center of the family time together allows other options in. Eating is just so darn easy! I heard Paula mention weekend trips to parks, mountain hikes, swimming at the lake, kite flying, bike riding .... how fortunate her kids were. They'd never come home with the scars overweight children and adolescents take. They may not even realize the iceberg they were steered away from, but Paula would know. and that's enough.

Her excitement was over the top as she fit back into clothes that were hanging in her closet for years. That excitement mounted when she came to meetings with stories of new clothes she was buying. WOW, I love that transition in members. To lose enough weight to move from the plus size department to the regular sizes is huge. It's far more than a simple walk from one section of the store to another. It represents something deeper. "I'm leaving the big people's section of the store forever. I'll never be there again unless I'm buying a gift for someone else, never again." Now a new first question would be on Paula's mind when she went to a store: 'what do I want' instead of 'what fits?' You can have a glorious time shopping for clothes in the cheapest store in the world. You can have a terrible time with a $500 gift card to the most expensive boutique in town. It ALL depends on how you feel about your size! Paula was reveling in the discovery of that.

Her casual style became her. I did see more youthful styles replace the oversized blouses. Tapered red leggings replaced elastic waist cloudy blue. More make-up and a bit of a bounce to her blond locks were all outer ways of expressing her happiness. They said to the world, "I like me enough to take care of me and I know I look great"

Paula making goal was not a surprise. Each week was just another step forward until the day she shrieked at the scale - I didn't need to run over, I knew what happened. Her family came to snap photos, applaud and cheer her on. I knew it would be for good. Consider it the safest bet I'd care to make. Knowing it's never over, Paula was there every week for the accountability of a weigh in. Sharing her struggles only made you admire her more and keep the class aware of the lifestyle change I'm always stressing. Paula was a triumph over her own hurdles, like all of us.

Most distressingly, her husband's job would force her to move out of the country. I was glad for her family. It was a 'too good to pass up' opportunity, it seemed. But, with such a brief time having Paula in the classes at goal - sigh - who knows how many others she would have mentored or inspired just by being her great self. She cried and I had to look away for a moment or I'd follow suit, when she told me how much I'd changed her life. How her kids were going to grow up to be slim, healthy, strong, happy, adventurous young people because of it. She was going to dance at all of their weddings in a size 8 dress. I believed every word of it.

Paula came back to visit one time. Showing up on a rare week when I wasn't there. Man, I hate that I missed her. I pumped the receptionist who did see her for details and I was delighted to know she'd gone right into the program where she lived and was still at her goal weight 5 years later. I could see the turnover in her head that she was ready to make the changes to reclaim her life from the day we'd met.

Paula, you are a true inspiration and it was my delight and privilege to know you.

TIPS: Paula lead her kids down a path of health with purpose! No 'but they need their treats' or 'but it's Halloween, they HAVE to have caramel apples' or 'they're skinny, it doesn't matter'. A great mother knows that their kids being thin has nothing do to with whether or not healthy eating is the rule of the home. It's a life skill.

TRAPS: Paula didn't fall into any, none at all, as close to perfect as I could know. Hey, sometimes it happens.

MONICA:

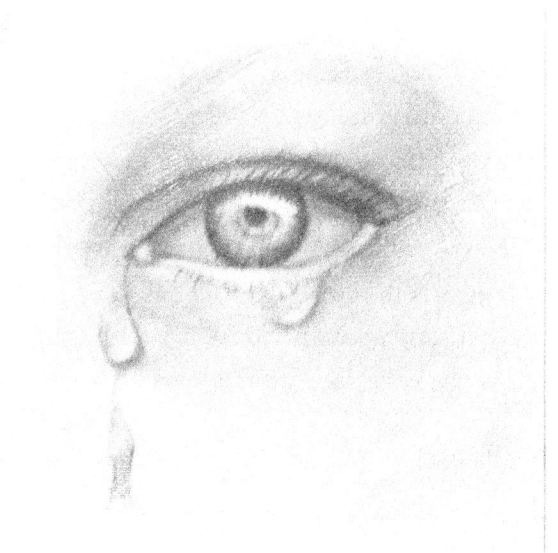

Monica and her mother joined my class as a smiling twosome with heart, willingness to learn and a genuine desire to follow the program and lose weight. It's a good thing, too. These helpful beginning states of mind would all be needed as both of these ladies were obese. Monica was at least 120# overweight while her mother - about 75/80. They were front row of class types that shared insightful observances about their own behavior and how they were turning their lives around. If you've ever spoken in front of a group before, you know how great it is having these kinds of people in your audience. They asked questions, shared on just about any topic I'd bring up. There was never any awkward quiet time when Monica and her mother were there: Dream members.

Monica's mother had not been a healthy eater and brought Monica up with the same habits. This was precisely my own experience. I identified with many of their stories and they, with mine. Most overweight kids had overweight parents. Not always, but it's the common thing. Life in their house was full of take out, home cooked meals of the highest fat and carb contents and plenty of sweets, too. No active time to counterattack it and, whom, another generation has the torch passed to them. Excuses were kept at a minimum, which I liked. Yes, Monica's mother was from a Midwestern town where they eat starch and meat and fry most of it and that's all she knew......but both were disgusted with their appearance and their health limitations enough to give their all to the program. I was proud of them.

I got the feeling Monica's mother was more there for her daughter. Granted, she, too, did need to lose weight. But the pounds on her child were more and she was most concerned for her. Without asking, I sensed that if she didn't come along, Monica wouldn't have, either. The embracing of the program was what I was so happy to see. The weight came off pretty regularly. Monica was literally discovering herself in her 20s in a way she was unable to before. Underneath layers of extra pounds was the woman she would become. I was always there to support them, but I served as more of an educator, really. Determination wasn't in short supply for them. On the rare occasion when Monica gained, she didn't mope or get defensive. She'd sometimes ask me to look at her journal to see if I could find any room for improvement. I loved how rational Monica was. It was paying off for her, well.

Self-esteem in young women is shaky. Self-esteem in overweight peo-ple is more so. Self-esteem for someone who was both is as vulnerable as it can get. Unless she was a very gifted actress, Monica didn't seem too bad off. She spoke of having friends. She went out. She looked you in the eye and her voice was articulate. She was groomed in her clothes, hair and make-up. All these are indications of someone who has self-esteem. So, if her foundation was this strong, I could only imagine how she'd blossom when her weight was shed.

I mention in class often that your weight loss slows as you approach goal. Monica, ever present in the classes, was ready when this hap-pened to her. She took the 1# losses with as much glee as the 3 and 4# losses she'd had at the start. It's just not realistic to expect those kinds of drops on a regular basis when you're no longer looking at 70+# anymore. And Monica wasn't. When she closed in on 100# off, I had the room give her the standing ovation she richly deserved. She cried, her mother cried, the room had criers - lots of emotions. Monica's mothers' own weight loss had stopped at about the half-way point. I'd been right, she was really there to support her kid and not interested in the work getting thin requires for herself. Well, I wouldn't push this. Monica had her whole life ahead of her. However, I'm very good with seniors, so I told her that if she ever changed her mind, I'd be there for her.

Clothes were a new joy for Monica. She would say that she'd long passed the smallest size she'd ever remembered being. Now, each new drop was a maiden voyage. Initially, she'd been thrilled to be a size 18. That meant no more 20s: again, a wise way to look at it. You can't go from 22 to a 12. The steps must be taken one at a time. XXL woman's blouses were being thrown out in the garbage. Size L was a moment she never even pined for because her faith wasn't even reaching that far. It was a delight to see this young lady do so well.

Then, the first chink in the picture: a vacation hadn't gone as well as expected. The time in another location without the routine they'd been thriving in was full of temptation and when the thread was let out, they let it spiral. But, they were at the next meeting and were ready to get back on track. Monica was within 20# of a goal weight range for her height. Onward, it was. As I've seen before, this vacation seemed to derail her much more than the week should have. Monica struggled. Gained weight, seemed unhappy when she'd come to classes (which she'd never done before), skipped weeks became common and big gains on the return. I sent postcards of concern and an offer of a discount on the fee for the missed time as an incentive to get them back. For a while, it worked. I was now worried for Monica. The euphoria period was over and the harsh glare from the heat crawling out of this slump brought was wearing on her. She'd lost so much. I wondered if she was getting prematurely complacent.

Boy, was I right. Sometimes members undo their good work by allowing themselves to accept a weight that is much less than what they used to be, but nowhere near thin. Their eyes don't perceive their bodies the way mine and others do. If they see the former size and then the new size, they see a huge difference. It's to be commended, but not become the very reason they don't make goal. I am in the 'get you thin business' not the get you 'thin-er business.' Too many compliments, too much success brought too much loosening up of the discipline and idling at the 15-yard line for Monica. Then, she dropped out.

But, not for good. When I saw her next, she was about 70# overweight again. Her mother was with her, too. She was rejoining, but with a new last name. Monica was married. Good for you, I exclaimed. She asked if he could come and see a class since he'd never been. Sure, I said. I met what might have been a truly nice man. But when I saw the dropped pants barely covering 1/2 his butt, the oversize jeans, the pot leaf shirt, the hung over looking eyes, doo rag gang looking, skinny as a stick figure with Monica, my poker face went on. Her healthy self-esteem may have been an impressive show. She could do so much better than this guy. I tried to maintain the appearance of a normal conversation with him. I wanted him to feel welcome. He was nice enough. But, I had a feeling he wasn't helping Monica. She may have been sold on the very first guy that had been nice to her. A common trap, girls with low self-esteem fall into. Flings are one thing; marriage is quite another. I wanted to ask Monica's mother if they'd known each other long, what did he do for a living, if he was supportive of her weight loss efforts ... but, I just didn't know how to tap dance around this. I didn't have to, turns out.

Monica's mother had said her husband didn't care if she was thin or fat and that's why she never got thin. Some people fall into a mindset of 'I'm married. So, it doesn't matter? Yes, it does. Not only because divorce is a very easy option, but because of your own health and self-worth. This is a sore subject with me, as you see. Well, after a couple of weeks with this guy sitting with his legs out stretched so I had to walk over them so as not to trip, she said it: "I'm married now to a wonderful man who doesn't care if I'm thin or fat." Just like her mother. Then he said something like, "Yea, fact is I'd rather she didn't worry about it so much. Then we could eat out more. She's always havin' to look stuff up and go through changes first." His speech was very mumbly, so this may not be a word for word exact quote, but it's close.

Poor Monica. Does she know what she's let happen to her? She'll be back one day, weighing who knows what, having to start over from square one, with or without her mother or this husband of hers. Maybe she'll look back with regret, maybe not. I know this, she'll get my 100% help. Monica, you're always welcome back.

TIPS: Seeing what's possible with success kept Monica focused. One size down at a time gets you from a 26 to a 12 better than bogus magic fixes. So, if you're in a class, hear what's being promised. Slow weight loss is going to be real world friendly. If you've established that this is a strong learning environment - ask and learn. Rarely did Monica come to classes without questions. Rarely did Monica leave classes without answers.

TRAPS: Getting a guy has unraveled so many women. Don't let this happen. BIGGER TRAP: If you're not thin, you're not finished. Think about someone who's never met you. They're unaware of your former size. They only see the 40# or so overweight person you are now. Not the 100+# person you recently were. While pictures can show a grand story, it's not the same. Rearrange your focus for continuous losing until it's all gone.

BETTY:

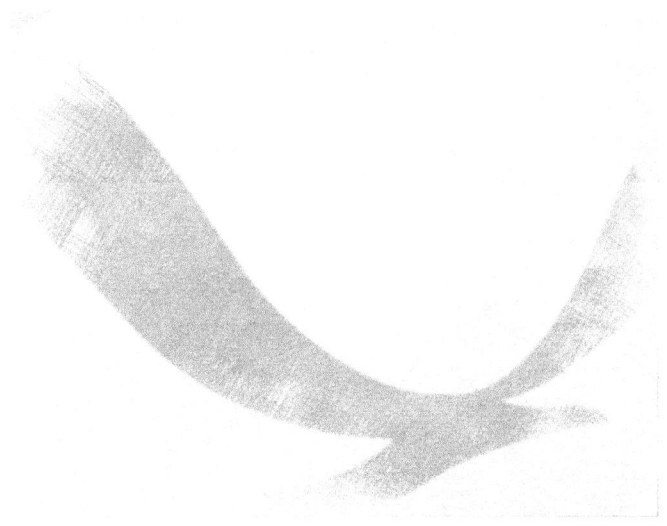

Betty was most people's mental picture of a sweet old lady: 70+, always smiling, congenial in mood, friendly to strangers, just an overall pleasant experience being around her. I met her at a satellite class we were running in a church. That place was chaos! Setting up for a meeting of over 100 bodies was a stressful ordeal that I went through for over 5 years. Lord, my car was so loaded with heavy cases of paper, scales, product and my own personal effects, I was afraid the alignment of my car would be damaged. Or, at least, it'd tip over like on the Flintstones when they order a dinosaur sized rack of ribs!

Folks like Betty made it worth it. She joined with her daughter. There were both more than 100# overweight. Her daughter seemed to be Betty's opposite. Depressed, quiet, quick to cry, misinterpret your intentions, unmotivated, sometimes awkward. How did Betty raise this child? Nature vs. nurture argument here, I suppose. Midwest transplants all the way. When I meet middle America raised types, I often hear about biscuits and gravy, meat loaf and gravy, cream chipped beef and gravy, corn beef hash and gravy, mashed potatoes aside just about everything and gravy, grits and gravy, barbecued pork and gravy, probably cereal and gravy. They like gravy! Butter can be occasionally substituted as a matter of taste. These kinds of foods have a devastating effect on the body. Obesity is only the most obvious. Betty and her daughter were no exceptions. Breathing trouble, inflamed joints, back pain, blood pressure medication and in Betty's case: full blown insulin dependent diabetes. Truly, her life was at risk.

Betty seemed to sense this. Health scares are a very common reason people join the program. The reality of what you are risking by overeating and carrying around dangerous amounts of extra pounds will eventually catch up with all of us. It's only a matter of when and how much the individual is willing to allow their own body to deteriorate before they draw the line. My own time drawing the line was ridiculously further down the road of damage than any sane or rational person would have taken. But, heck, the first thing I'll admit was that sanity and rational thinking were 2 things I lacked in regards to food. So, there!

I understand people like that. Unfortunately, field research has shown that joining the program as a knee jerk reaction to a health scare has a notoriously short shelf life. Time eases the blow and fear wears off some. Then, the poor habits that got you into the mess return. I've seen this happen quite often. I am persistent yet patient with this. I caution joiners in that position against it. At least the early warning may help some avoid hitting that iceberg.

Betty listened at each meeting, shared well, lost weight, participated in whatever type of interaction I was trying to get the class to do: a model member. The room bonded with her and as her weight loss climbed to very impressive numbers, her glowing reports began to include lessening of her insulin prescription. Her goal - 100% off it. I cannot tell you how much I wanted to see Betty achieve this.

Meanwhile, her daughter was polar opposite. Never losing much of anything, each week, a glum excuse wielding card was pulled out of the rolodex for why this week it was impossible for her to do it. Of course, I listen when members go this route, but I do not let them off the hook. I would be a terrible teacher if I did. I challenge them to rise above the reliance on the old fall backs. I point out that they are chiefly responsible for their starting weight and will not help them. I helped write the excuse rolodex, so I can criticize it.

Worst of all, every week Betty moved forward, her daughter would cry and hang her head down. I know part of it was shame from watching this older woman with more obstacles than her succeed right next to her. But I was greatly concerned that her glum, woe is me routine might make Betty feel guilty and she'd go into mother mode and stop losing weight and saving herself to make her daughter feel better. Happily, Betty did not fall into that trap. When her weight loss went past 100#, I had a certificate printed up for her to commemorate the accomplishment and the whole room stood up and cheered her with thunderous applause. And yes, her doctor took her entirely off of her insulin. She is a hero of mine.

Question, dear reader: Is anyone who makes goal finished? Cured? Doesn't need to attend classes anymore? No, no and no. The biggest mistake people who lose all their weight make is to immediately stop doing the very things that got them there. I have witnessed this over and over through the years. Maintaining your weight is perpetual care. Like taking care of a garden is. There isn't a certain amount of gallons of water you can count where grass will forever remain green after. Like grass, bushes, flowers.... if one takes it on, they are accepting that it will be a forever commitment. Weight loss is the same. Be prepared to make only changes while you're losing weight that you can accept that you'll be doing on a permanent basis. Anything else will make your odds of keeping it off lower. Betty kept attending and her weight stayed down for a while. Then, she went to the hospital for an unrelated matter and had to be on medical leave. When she returned, she'd put some weight back on. She made NO excuses. During her convalescence she just couldn't exercise. Oh, yes, let me add more to the list of Betty's positive and amazing feats. She found out what activity she could do despite being limited and water aerobics became a way of life for her. See, some people see obstacles and sit, stagnate and wait for it or somebody else to move them. Others find ways to go around them. She was losing the weight again when she informed me that, sadly, she was moving back to the Midwest. I was heavy hearted to hear it. I don't know if she will have a support system in gravy-land to continue. If they're like her daughter, it's unlikely.

I hope if I'm graced with as many years on this Earth as Betty has had, I'm as positive, brave and open minded as her. A great lady.

TIPS: Health is wealth. Betty believed her grim health was changeable and, therefore, it changed. The large majority of all obstacles are conquerable. Can't do this exercise, what about that one? Can't drive, where's a ride? On meds, what needs to happen to wean off them? Betty checked off a list of wars waged on her body's conditions and won! You'd be wise to do the same.

TRAPS: Betty is another platinum star that didn't do too much of anything wrong. All I can add is a restatement of what's been said. Are you living with what doesn't need to be lived with?

PAUL:

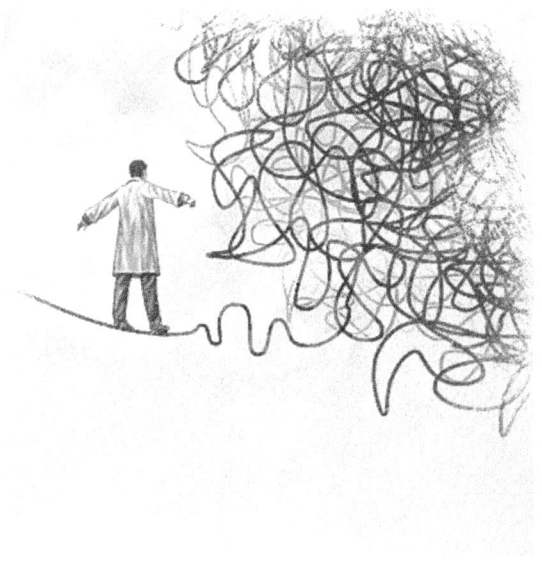

I must state right up front regarding this story – it is one person's side that I have no way to verify. It's about a man named Paul who's chance at weight loss was undone by his wife. I know there are always two sides to stories like this, so I am prefacing it with what I observed and what was told to me.

I met Paul when I took a class over from a teacher who'd gotten another job. Teacher changes are met with resistance by some students. I've been on both sides of that. After a couple of classes, I'd won this one over well, I must say. Paul came up to me to tell me he was glad they had me in the room. I'm always glad when students let me know I'm doing well by them. Paul was my age, height, build and hair color. We could be related. He was a gregarious guy, too. Another trait I like in both men and women. He was down 60+# already and was going to get the 35 / 40# remaining off with me. This would be a 100# loser. Great, let's do this.

Paul was a gold standard member. A front seat sitter who always had well thought out questions, paid attention, was willing to change and was already reaping tremendous benefits from the weight already gone. There was no doubt he'd make goal - this was a freight train going to Slimsville (I love when spell check questions my many intentional puns). Indeed, Paul was at goal w/a bright future ahead of him. He was likable, had many friends and was eager to keep working to maintain his loss.

We spoke before and after meetings often and both shared a desire to have a work out partner to keep us accountable and motivate each other. We shared a hit and miss gym history and both saw the potential benefit to us making that a commitment. Problem was we lived on totally opposite sides of town and our work schedules were as incompatible as could be. Darn it. One time, Paul asked if we could have a one-time work out after a meeting. I'd shared with the room I worked with a personal trainer and could pass on many useful tips to any interested member. Sure, next week we'd plan on it. We had a good workout: warm up, calisthenics, weights, cardio.... timing together. We both would have done well with that accountability and camaraderie.

Fate blessed Paul soon with a pretty lady who became his wife. A tall attractive woman who joined the program to lose 30# or so and I enjoyed her company. She followed the program well and made goal in a rather quick time. This isn't always a good thing. We advocate slow losses in the program for many reasons. One is simply you need practice for the task of learning how to eat differently for the rest of your life. A way of eating you've done for a few months just isn't enough practice. Paul's new wife had lost weight, yes, but seemed to approach it as a diet. Soon after goal, she wasn't attending anymore.

Soon, children came. Soon, Paul's weight began going up again. Paul shared his frustrations with me. His wife was from the South and had Southern habits. Her cooking was good and she earned money with her culinary skills, too. He was unable to resist the foods he'd smell when he got home from work. I always emphasize how crucial a clean house is to keep you doing the right thing.

But, Paul said that wasn't going to happen. Her habits were in her soul and her love of cooking wasn't going to be altered or interrupted by him. It was his problem.

Paul's weight went over 100+# again = back to where he'd been and then more. He came to classes sweaty, tired looking and quite defeated. Nevertheless, he'd try and smile and make pleasant small talk through his pain. I admire that trait in anyone and try to conduct myself that way, too. Privately, I'd ask him what was going on. I thought of him as a genuine friend and this conversation was to be without a class listening in. He'd hesitate and I would ask about the family dining situation. He'd say his wife made food for every occasion and there was always baking, frying, cooking and massive portions in their kitchen. She had put a few pounds back on, but not all of it. She'd been cooking like this her entire life and was used to it. Perhaps this was part of where her will power came from. If she could do it, he should be able to. I suggested he make something else to eat. If she wanted to prepare her food one way, he could bring home sandwiches from Subway or microwave a light frozen meal. Evidently, he'd tried that and it caused trouble. She'd spent all day cooking and he wasn't going to eat it. Or more insultingly, bring something else!

"Happy wife, happy life", I hear it said. So, Paul didn't object, but didn't have it in him to resist. All his weight back on also brought the health troubles with it you could predict. Paul was a devoted father and took his kids to the park, coaches their little sports teams, golfs with his buddies (but takes the cart again while he'd proudly said he was walking the entire course with ease when he was at goal) and eats his wife's food. He was stuck. There was nothing he could do. His objections only caused arguments and his wife was implacable on this. Until his kids are grown, this would likely not change.

I hear too many stories about unsupportive spouses and the damage they cause. Most of students are women, so it's usually men that are the villain in the story. Like my intro said, I don't know the whole story and do know there are two sides and maybe the tales my female members are telling me are colored to their advantage and edited. That's likely and it's likely in Paul's case, too. But, I do believe his dilemma was genuine. He'd been as glowing, proud and happy a man who was ready to party and take on the world as I'd seen in the program when he made goal. If he's not leaving his wife, he would have to dig down deep for the strength to overcome the living situation he's in. But he's a combination of unwilling and surrendered to his fate. He speaks of his perpetual back pain often. He is a ticking time bomb for a heart attack, stroke, diabetes, falls, joint troubles and a laundry list of more.

I don't know how true what Paul's told me is. But, if it is, I hesitate as I write this, shame on her. Shame on ALL people who are not willing to change or support the person they claim to love in this. You make it so much harder on them and my job harder, too. Your position is so valuable. You have a chance to be the co-pilot that encourages, listens, changes with your spouse, allows your own life and routine to, yes, maybe need to get rearranged some. Isn't that what love is?

A toast: to all the glorious husbands and wives and partners that walk the walk with us. You make us happy with your proof that you care. You may need to lose weight, too and will benefit from the healthy food habits or just want to see your sweetheart do well and are glad to contribute in whatever ways you can. You don't put us down for our lack of your will power. You are not threatened by increased self-esteem in your partner meaning they'll leave you. You want to be a united defense when others try to overtake you. You are a true hero in this - all of you. You'll reap many rewards from a woman who's thin and has her confidence back. She won't forget your co- operation. Paul's struggle continues.

TIPS: If you need the power of 2 or a group to keep consistent on a self-improvement project, do it. Some thrive best if someone else is expecting them to show up. They've arranged their own day around the same thing. Activities that cannot be done without 2 keeps some more accountable.

TRAPS: I'm a weight loss counselor, not a marriage counselor. I've seen many members undo fantastic work via spouses. I invite your input on how you're turned this dilemma into a positive if you've faced it.

EVE:

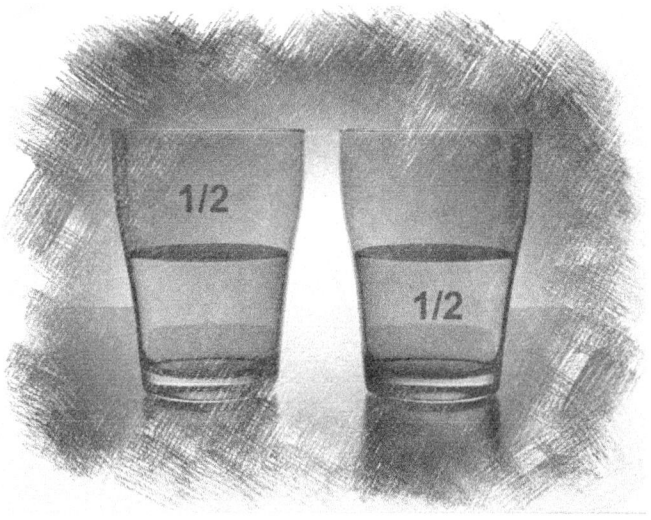

Regarding the perks of weight loss, I must admit I don't understand people who don't care about their appearance. I draw huge strength from my love of being thin, feeling attractive, wearing stylish clothes and knowing I can buy anything I want in any clothing store because I don't buy anything I want in the bakery. If I truly didn't care about my looks, where would my motivation come from? For those who are not bothered by their lack of care in basic presentable dressing or even hygiene, what is it? - Health?

It would seem so. As much as I like to joke about my superficial glee I am in daily regarding the surface platinum benefits of being slim (I am deeply shallow, I like to say), health is wealth. Without it, you don't have a lot. I was very, very lucky my years of morbid obesity didn't kill me or disable me or leave me with scars or handicaps that could easily have happened and would have negatively impacted my quality of life no matter what I weigh. I pushed that envelope foolishly too many years and am one of the healthiest middle aged men I know. I am very lucky.

Eve was not so lucky. Eve had suffered a stroke that left her with permanent damage. I have observed when tragic things like this take place people react in one of two ways - they bitterly retreat and morph into a 'professional sick person' who's rage about their fate cripples their ability to feel joy and happiness in anything anymore. Substance abuse and depression often follow and there they remain. While other people gravitate towards positivity and tackle the challenges with a determination to lead as regular a life as they can. These types go to rehab, struggle but persevere, overcome obstacles and modify their existence in all ways they must and keep living. These are the heroes I'd hope I follow in their footsteps if I'm ever required to.

Eve was 80# overweight, 40 something and as sweet as can be. She spoke slowly, struggling with certain pronunciations and used her hands expressively to convey thoughts well. It was no trouble communicating with her. You paid more attention, which is a lost art in our fast paced technology driven society. I found her delightful, brave, and refreshing from our first meeting. She could do this!

Taking notes worked well for Eve and she contributed to the classes and isn't shy. She made fast friends with other members, had insightful things to share and was also as human as all of us are with her struggles. Candy bars and sweets were her downfall. She was addicted to them. I knew I recognized a fellow comrade in her. I used to have a 4 to 5 candy bar a day habit. I am as addicted to candy bars as I was as a kid. When I go to convenience stores, I stare at them wistfully: remembering their chocolate-y, carmel-y, nutty, gooey yumminess and get nostalgic. I can't un-remember what they taste like. Then I remember the damage and I go buy gas.

I always included Eve in classes fully and why not? She was no victim. It took her a bit longer to speak, but her bravery and good attitude were often referred to by me for the excuse makers that she'd trumped their reason for why they didn't lose weight that week. As her achieved milestones like 50# off, 10, 20 and 30% of her starting weight off - she beamed with happiness. Her only trouble was the expense her constant need for smaller clothes was causing. What a problem, right?

She came to class one day with her hair very short. I asked her why she'd cut it so short. She said it was being donated to women with cancer. I nearly cried. After an embrace, I told her she would be the type to do this. She expected no sympathy from anyone and leads as normal a life as she can. I say this not only to fully involve the reader in her glorious positivity, but also because she had the regular expected snags, too.

As often happens, when members get ½ to 2/3 of their weight off, the margin for error narrows. Their discipline must increase. She'd been losing so well; we didn't have too many out of meeting detailed talks about her day to day eating because there was no need. Eve was doing fine. Then, the wall: the wall hit by anyone who loses to that percentile - a spectacular year followed by a stagnant one. Eve reached out in frustration. Her note taking had served her well here.

She had records of most of her eating that I could peruse to find what I could. Glad to put in the extra time - for any member, but one as special as Eve - even more so.

Wow, what I saw. Eve had lost her weight up to that point eating nearly all processed food and candy. While her portions had been reasonable, the nutritional values were lacking. Eve was a life-long hater of cooking and never got the skill. I don't cook too much, either. Day after day was full of crackers, puddings, frozen dinners, rolls and candy. Well, this was clearly what had happened. I had to inform Eve that this wouldn't do anymore. She seemed chagrined, but didn't protest since she knew it was true. That didn't mean she had to be glad of it, though.

We're in the process of rewiring Eve. This is very difficult after many years. I feel its lure daily and must fight it, so I understand. I say to joiners, I didn't get thin because I woke up one day and suddenly Hershey bars didn't taste good anymore. They're wonderful. There's nothing like the face of this adult man eating a Hershey bar! A Hershey bar, no. More like me eating 3 or more. I stay away from them because I don't have it in me to eat one. Eve had to make this decision for herself. But, I will try to tip the scale in favor of what I know needs to happen for her to take off the additional weight.

Eve's load to bear had been higher than most peoples. She's taken on so much and now; I'm asking her to give up something she loves. No one wants to hear this, but it's what I must do. This assimilation is going on as I type this. But, my faith that Eve will rise to this occasion is high. I am only thinking of a way to get what her favorite flower is casually in a conversation somehow. Then, I'll know what kind of bouquet to have on hand for her when she makes goal.

TIPS: When you're not losing, reach out and have written records. I speak for just about anyone who'll be looked to help dig you out of any plateau. Eve got quick optimum help due to that very thing.

TRAPS: You can't expect thin with no rearranging of the healthy - unhealthy ratio tipping to the former in a big way. 80 / 20 seems reasonable if you exercise. If you won't, the ratio decreases. All actions have consequences. Make wise choices.

KIDS:

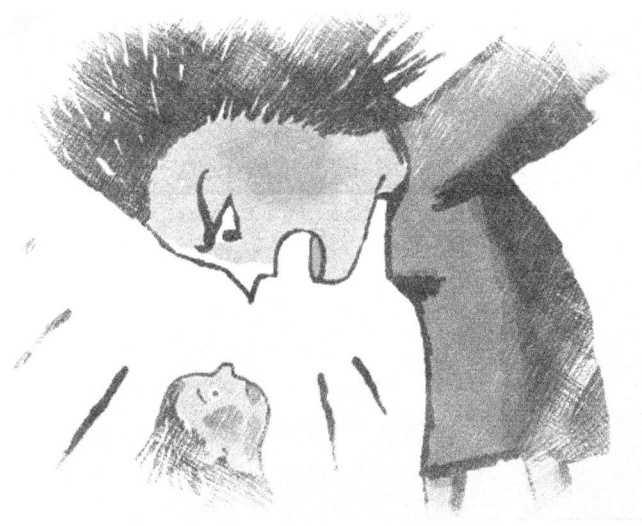

I was an overweight child. Food was my primary passion from my earliest memory. A famous family story is that soon after my birth, I wouldn't stop crying. No matter what my mother tried, it didn't end. In a fit, I was brought to the doctor. After relieving them that nothing was medically wrong, he said, "This boy's hungry!" Some watered down farina was put to my mouth and, like magic, the noise ends. I opened my mouth to maximum ability to indicate, "YAYYYYY! More, please. Make it snappy."

Being overweight while growing up was touched upon in my intro-duction. Simply, it was awful. The obesity epidemic was decades away. The 'fat kids' were the few and the marked for teasing. Now, the pandemic of childhood obesity has plagued the nation. The heart-breaking ripple effects are grim. For the first time in America's history, the next generation is less healthy and likely to live shorter lives than their parents. So sad. So tragic.

In the course of teaching classes, I meet some of these cases. Often good intentions are not applied correctly by the worried parents. The core of the healing requires a family united effort to turn around unhealthy behaviors that will save the minor. I have not seen this happy ending as often as I'd like. An overweight minor simply plopped in our laps with a "fix them" request, that doesn't do.

CASE #1: I only saw this young man one time. He was 16. Not particularly overweight. But his mother and grandmother were very concerned. When I introduced myself to him and stuck out my hand, he held his head down and didn't reply. His mother and grandmother treated me to a list of his shortcomings. All the effort they were putting into him, what he wasn't doing and so on. I tried to focus on him and treat him like a proper young man. He was interrupted and when he did speak, it was so quietly I had to lean forward to make it out. At his weigh in, they hovered all over him. Asked what he weighed, if it wasn't to their liking…he hadn't lost weight. They were ticked. I felt so sorry for him. I was a newer teacher and if that were today, I would have spoken more sternly to them. "Back off!" is what they had coming to them. His manhood was wrecked. I am certain that if this was the standard atmosphere he was reared in, then his personal development was stifled to a point that extensive therapy would be needed. He stumbled out with the nitpicking on both sides of his head going non-stop.

CASE #2: A thin, good looking step mother brought in her step daughter who was about 12 or 13 years old. I never met the father. She was also not too overweight. Puberty isn't a smooth transition for any of us. She seemed overwhelmed with the program experience. It isn't easy for adults to make the lifestyle adjustments, let alone a 13-year-old. It can only happen at that age if there's smooth collective co-operation. Her weigh-ins were also hovered over and when the desired progress wasn't what was expected, she was berated. She got told how she was wasting her step mother's money, time and effort. She, too, was following the 'diet' and was dropping pounds. Pounds that she didn't even need to lose because she was already thin, thank you. It was just to prove how easy it was and what a failure she was. I tried to council them in a diplomatic way about the counter-productive outcome that we were dealing with. How do I say, 'frankly, I think you're the problem, ma'am.'? They did not stay around too long. Now, she is a young adult and I can only imagine how she looks back at the experience she endured.

CASE #3: So sad! I have said here that co-operation with the adults is a basic essential for success dealing with overweight minors. They make many decisions for the household. They spend the money. They buy the groceries. They have a disproportionate amount of power, which is as it should be. However, that carries responsibility with it. When couples break up that have a child, the child is a connection that will keep them in each other's company. Therefore, a civil relationship is needed for the child's sake. I met a 12-year-old boy that weighed in at over 280. He did not speak above a whisper, kept his head down and didn't seem to engage in a single thing that was going on in the room. His mother was with him. After paying, she informed me she was not staying. I tried to persuade her otherwise. I was told that his father would be picking him up and that is was the start of his visitation time. I was told he was diagnosed with diabetes and had heart palpitations. Neither of his parents had a history of it. I asked this so I could rule out inherited factors. It was solely a result of his morbid obesity. I tried to tell her that the program would not work without involvement of the adults he lives with. A brisk 'Good Luck' was given me as she said she had to leave. He was on his own.

After the meeting, during which he sat in a comer, spoke not a word and seemed to be daydreaming, I sat down to try to reach him. I had not pointed him out during the meeting as I felt it would terrify this young man. He held his head down and I could not reach him in any relevant way, despite my best efforts. When his father arrived, I asked if I could speak privately to him. I hoped there would be a different reaction form him than from his mother. He was just the same. He was busy with work, it wasn't his fault he was so fat, his mother was a _____ and he was sure as _____ not going to take the time to learn the program for the sake of his son. They left in silence. I stood there in dismay. They were frankly allowing him to die a slow, painful death. I can't even delve into the mental damage this boy was suffering. He was in need of so much assisted help from a physician, a counselor specializing in family therapy and a weight loss plan with a long term, easy to follow design that would help avoid the serious health disintegration surely in front of him. None of this happened. He was dropped off by one or the other parent for the next few weeks. He was left off without the correct payment since neither parent had bothered to read the material he'd been provided with or knew what it cost. I waived the fee when the receptionist called me over. He never lost weight and I never got invited into his trust. It was too late for it to be that easy. After about six weeks, I never saw him again.

CASE #4: In some areas, the classes happen in libraries, churches, social centers. Anyplace that may not merit enough business to set up a permanent center. The set-up, break down and display of the meeting means we have scales that can be transported. The top weight limit is lower than the scales in many centers. They're too heavy for staff to carry them around. It was in this exact type of meeting I met Lourdes, a red headed, 15-year-old. She was more self-assured than the other cases I've discussed. She'd taken the bus and arrived on her own. But she wasn't confused or seemed afraid to speak to adults. I liked her immediately. She was so overweight, I was worried she was over the scale's limits. They go to 440.I knew she was over that. After she filled out the registration form, paid and stepped on - sure enough - it flat lined. This has only happened to me a few times. It's always SO sad. But, I always try to diffuse the situation as diplomatically and sensitively as I can. Most people expected it. We have only a couple of options. One of them is they cannot attend a satellite class. They must go to a proper center where the scale will accommodate them. Or they have to go to where they have loading dock scales and have a signed note verifying their weekly weight until it gets to a number we can manage. Lourdes took the news with amazing maturity. Not surprised and even aware of what she'd need to do. She was used to being obese. She knew where she would go to be weighed. After we spoke, she traced us back through some of her experience. Parental neglect doesn't even begin to describe it. 500# at 15, she'd hit 400 at 13, was 300 at 11, 200 at 8, 100 at 6 .... tragic. Her story was embellished by my co-worker after Lourdes left. I was full of sorrow for her, admiration for her, anger at the people who allowed this to happen. I did not live in the area, but my co-worker did. She said she lived in a trailer park and had been allowed to eat gargantuan amounts of junk food from birth. They had had local authorities inspect their living circumstances before and Lourdes' room was found to be full of doughnut boxes and pizza boxes piled all over. Evidently, she was eating dozens of them and whole pies at one sitting all her life. They were always just above legal requirements to not be quarantined.

Her weight was coming off. I was encouraged. Then, she was not attending. When I saw her one more time, she came over to thank me for all I'd done. School was going to not allow her to come to classes anymore. After school activities and studies had to come first. She was very grateful. I didn't know what to think. I was amazed she took place in after school activities. She even seemed to have friends and rather healthy self-esteem. Lourdes was very impressive. I know trying to do the program on one's own rarely works out. I was not optimistic. Fast forward a few years. I am in a grocery store and I run into Lourdes! Tall, teenage red heads tend to stick in one's mind. Besides, I'm amazingly good at remembering faces and names. She was considerably slimmer! Not slim, but at least ½ of her extra weight less than when we'd met. She seemed happy to see me, too. She'd had gastro intestinal bypass surgery as soon as she'd turned 18, the legal minimum. She was the type of case that surgery was made for. It isn't magic. I have members who've had that and other various surgical eating restrictions that are not any substitute for your own need to manage what you eat. She was in life threatening danger and it was very necessary. She was in college, was losing weight and said she never forgot the program and how we helped her believe in herself. I was smiling all day after that.

I could have added many more cases. But, I've made the point. If the parents are not willing to cooperate and be taught themselves, it's very unlikely the minor will be able to dig out of their situation. Determined types like Lourdes are the exception to the rule. It's my particular desire to give extra care and time to anyone who walks in with overweight children. It reminds me of me and my mother. She did her best. She was not fully in control of her own eating habits and her inconsistency with what was cooked and served did neither of us any good. I was so unwilling to help myself that even if she were in a better position to lead, it would likely not have worked. That's my failure. But, it fuels my vigilance to steer families suffering to recovery. It takes family power.

TIPS: Parents must be involved! I expect less leading of the journey from minors. Too many variables are out of their hands. Don't give the burden to them. They need you to take this on at the same level of commitment that they'll be at.

TRAPS: Parents must not smother, either. Supportive and overbearing are not the same things. Also, some kids know how to manipulate very well. Be fine-tuned to this and don't take any nonsense from them.

FUNNY MOMENTS:

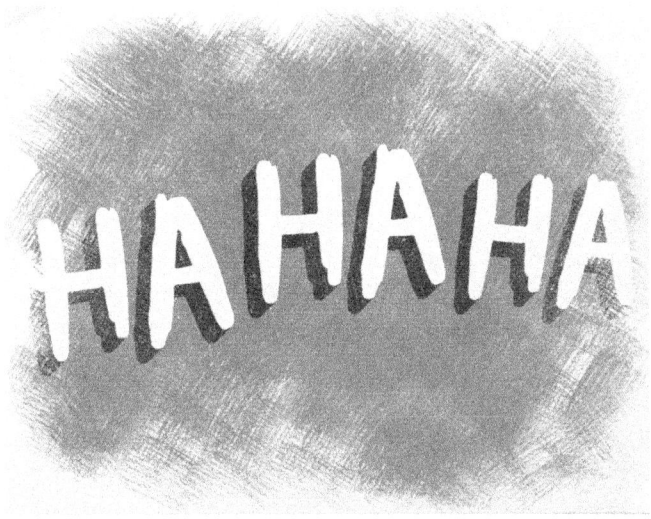

It's true, the cliché, "You couldn't have made that up." All of the following stories, comments, and anecdotes really happened in classes of mine exactly how they're described. Hope they make you laugh.

1— A member asked me, 'Can wine coolers count as fruit? I wanted to say, 'Yes'. I could imagine her staggering down the street, drunk, saying: 'They say at leassss 5 a day.... for my health.'

2— I love chocolate so much my husband has to hide the Ex-Lax.

3— I was asked if sex counted towards exercise. Without missing a beat, I said, 'If you do it right.'

4— I want to lose enough to see my taco. (it took me a moment to realize what she'd meant!)

5— A baby in my class farts. A rather loud one, I must say. At times like this, you have to improvise and think on your feet. I decided to test the room. I said, 'Did that baby just fart?' The class roared with laughter. Confirmation they're relieved I'd brought it up. They were bottled up with trying to be mature adults and not laugh. So, one step further, I say, "and the guy behind them said, 'Oh, thank goodness, he blamed it on the baby!" They laughed even louder.

6— A woman asked my receptionist if she could re-weigh after she took a dump.

7— On a bet, a member was ½# away from a $100 bet. I said, was there anything she could remove to lighten the number. After thinking briefly, she took out her dentures and won the Benjamin.

8— Rediscovering your body as you lose weight is a very exciting process. However, it can be confusing. One member said when she first felt her pelvis, she thought she'd broken a bone and it was protruding.

9— My husband told me I dress too sexy for my work - so I quit my job!

10— After a long night and a 25-minute orientation, a new member told me she hadn't been listening to anything I said and I needed to repeat it – all of it.

11— I don't want to lose my extra weight because one day should I ever get cancer I want a lot of fat for me to live upon.

12— In the store, I'd eaten so many cookies while I was still shopping, I couldn't face the checker with what was left. So, I put the package behind the toilet paper and walked quickly to the next aisle.

13— With all the fiber I'm eating, my kids call me the fart machine.

14— Without my gut, my pants all need hemmed. I thought I'd shrunk. Amazing what a flat tummy does!

15— A lady is married to an avid golfer. She shares enthusiastically at meetings. I wanted her to tell us one of her rituals, she said, 'For luck, before I come here, I kiss my husband's balls.' She shrieked when she saw people's reactions. 'His GOLF balls! His GOLF balls!' I've never seen a redder face!

16—An acquaintance told me she'd seen my husband in public with another woman. I was delighted to tell her it was me!

17— Self-esteem growth is a huge pay off of losing weight. One lady around the age of 50 said her husband is always getting on her case about wanting her in good enough shape to wear a bikini and look good in it. Now that I feel better about myself, I looked him in the eye and shot him an 'After you fit in and look good in a Speedo, bud.' He never brought it up again.

18— My grandkid said his parents and he went bed shopping. When he laid on the waterbed, he told the salesman and my son-in-law and daughter that it felt like grandma's belly. OUCH! But, it got me to join!

19— My fiancé has a fetish for big women. He told me he didn't want a skinny wife. No problem. Now he doesn't have a skinny girlfriend, either.

20— As a life-long remover of size revealing labels and tags, I now wear clothes that I'm not embarrassed to have anyone know the number. But, I never knew how dang itchy they are! They drive me crazy.

21— Good food being all that's allowed in my house got my unhealthy eating, sloppy and overweight relatives out of mine and into hotels when they visit now - YEAAAII!

22— I used to be a showgirl until I got IBS, now I can't dance. Too risky: it loosens stool. - Great to know!

23— When you speak in public, you HAVE to expect the unexpected. As I talked, a man in the back row stuck his index finger so far up his nose, it disappeared. GROSS! I spontaneously laughed. Students wondered why I laughed. With no desire to embarrass the guy, I instantly connected a humorous aside to what I'd been saying and we moved on. It's a good skill to have. Inside, I wanted to ask him if he was scratching his brain!

24— A man from another class came out of the bathroom in just his underwear to weigh. Shocked, I verified he was, indeed, in his skivvies. I told him, 'Sir, you're in public. You can't weigh in just in your underwear. They're women here.' He stared at me like he didn't get what the big deal was, got dressed and left and I never saw him again.

25— Having submitted 2 weeks of journals for me to investigate, a frustrated member that insisted he was doing program correctly eagerly awaited my advice. I saw days of fried food, nuts, cheese, nothing being weighed or measured properly. When I asked what his take on this stubborn plateau he was on might be, he said, 'I think I'm overdoing fruit.'

26— A woman joined, grabbed all of our information books and said she wasn't returning or had any interest in staying for the meeting or talking to me at all. She told me she's a psychic and uses our program to give her 'diagnosis' to her obviously gullible clientele. Magic, right!

27— A morbidly obese woman walks in to join. Using a walker, breathing very heavily, head and shoulders hunched over, taking baby steps. She gets to the counter, says she needs to lose weight and has a very tough job. I ask, 'What job is that?' She says, 'I'm a home health care nurse and I assist the infirm and disabled.' I nearly fell over. I pity any post-operative person she's assigned to.

28— ROOKIE ERROR ON MY PART: I wouldn't leave myself off this list. In my first month working on my own, I'm in a class and we're connecting very well. Somehow, Michael Jackson comes up in conversation. In doing an impression of his moves, I briefly grab my crotch. One of my mentors had been there to check me out. After the meeting, she said, 'Don't do that again?' It was sound advice and I took it to heart. While you can relax to a certain point with a group, you must keep one eye on yourself and not get too caught up in any given moment.

29— Every week, this guy would come to meetings after teaching a Zumba class. He was extremely proud that he was a certified Zumba instructor. That was fine. What wasn't fine was that every week, he got up to the scales, bent over to remove his shoes (slowly) and treated all those behind him to a view of his behind. No plumber joke could prepare you for his obviously not wearing underwear moon view. People would gawk, laugh, turn away....as their pleasure dictated. He seemed utterly oblivious to this. Week in and week out, no matter what time of day, a crack of the moon was forecasted.

30— True story: I once had a man join a noon class that was - very - clearly - drunk. Eyes at 1/2 mass, slurring his words drunk. He'd been the only joiner and I spent about 30 minutes explaining the program to him which was a complete waste of time. He took the material and staggered out. I have often thought of him awakening with a horren-dous hangover and seeing all the debris at his bed. He looks down at it and says, 'I joined a diet club? I gotta quit drinking.' He is at his first AA meeting and he tells of his rock bottom moment. Around him are tough guys who speak of getting tattooed with regrettable images, waking up in the gutter, marrying someone they don't even know, getting into fights that land them in jail...and his horrific tale begins, 'I joined a diet group.'

31— First leader I ever met told a true tale I'll close with: Thinking her husband was away for a few hours, she'd drawn herself a bath and surrounded the tub with Oreos. Her plan was to wash something, have a cookie, wash something, have a cookie. Chocolate-y bliss! As you can guess, husband comes home earlier than expected. In a panic, she sweeps all the Oreos into the water. It was the only option. As they melted into a black sludge all around her, her husband looked at her and said, 'Wow, you're dirty. What were you doing?'

PROLOGUE - THE PLAN:

Good intentions. They can spark a fire. This is exhilarating and fills us with hope and the promise of a soon to be better future. Ain't no stoppin' me now!

Then, what? Good intentions go so far. You wake up like a dream has ended. Maybe you can't fully explain why, but you know the fire is out or very near out. It happens frequently: not to you, not this time. You're going to keep your fire burning naturally and not converting to artificial presto logs. This requires a plan, a good plan. Blueprints for a good plan are what you're about to read.

In the first year, everything is new. There are so many firsts, trials and potential to have fire replaced by Stern-0 and then by icy indifference. I've arranged 4 time periods into top 10 lists. It's a familiar format. It's easily absorbed. The 10 are not in any 'best to worst' order. They're commonly, collectively to be expected phases numerous people go through. I've counselled many through them to victory. The intervals of time may happen at varying stages, they're only approximations. Some are in your control to schedule (such as photo taking) and some are not. It's likely they'll all occur in your year one.

What's more important - the action steps being offered. Some of you may decide after reading them that they're just basic common sense. Anyone could do this and get thin on attempt #1. There's nothing Earth shattering. Well, recall, I offered you no miracle, Earth shattering new discoveries. But, most people DON'T get thin (at attempt #1, next to none). So, there is a barrier in the path. Here is where I wanted to step in and offer useful interference. Read and re-read what's in 'The Plan'. Far too many people have not achieved their goals and delay for years by lacking basic tools (a plan). Prepare for your life to soon be exceptionally better. You're getting thin, staying that way and never using the word 'diet' again!

THE PLAN AT 7 DAYS:

1— RELEIF / PANIC: Congratulations, you've made a very wise decision. You're going to lose weight and keep it off. The road will not be easy, but the reward is beyond price. How do you feel? It's often a combination of relief (whew, I can begin to reclaim my life again) and / or panic (boo hoo, no more tasty food). While you'll discover that you will not have to give up any specific food, you will need to scale back some. You gotta give to get! It's ON!!

2— TAKE A PHOTO: As neutral a background as possible and neutral clothing. This is not a photo that needs to be shared, it's for you. This is the start of a collage, a pictorial keepsake of your transformation.

3— TAKE YOUR MEASUREMENTS: This is a scary one for some people. Yes, the first ones sting. But, please believe this - you'll want the information later on. Get someone you love and trust or do them yourself, but do it! Don't have a tape measure, they're 99 cents at most pharmacies. Measure your neck, chest, waist, and hips. If you're more ambitious, measure your thighs and how far out your belly at its widest is from the floor, bring the tape measure down and see how much space there is between there and the tip of your toes. One day, you'll look down and see them again!

4— DEJUNK YOUR HOME: It's logical. When you're tempted, you can't eat what isn't there. You know the kryptonite that needs to go. My definition of kryptonite for our purposes is: fattening foods you're legitimately incapable of having around you and not overeating. Only to be eaten out now when you're being watched and portions are restricted. Allow this to sink in. It's 100% logical. If you are trying to quit smoking, there should be no cigarettes in your home, right? If you're trying to quit drinking, no alcohol in the home makes perfect sense. If you're trying to quit gambling, no casino visits - it's a toxic place for you. It's the same principle.

5— BUY A FOOD SCALE: Many overweight people have completely out of whack ideas about portions. Don't fool yourself for a minute thinking you can 'guesstimate' portions. You can't! This makes you normal, so embrace it. Be prepared for lots of 'sticker shock' when confronted with reality realizations. THIS is 4 ounces of meat - WOW. THIS is a cup of pasta - WHOA. THIS is 2 tablespoons of salad dressing - THAT EXPLAINS A LOT. You get the idea. No wonder you weigh what you weigh. It's a necessary tool. Measuring cups, bowls and spoons are extremely helpful, too. Don't leave your success to chance!

6— DOCUMENT EATING: Yes, write it all down. Writing makes it real. Many overweight people have serious denial regarding their eating. This journey will require reading and writing. The information keeps you honest and will save time later. KEEP all written food diaries. As time goes on, they'll prove invaluable. Trust me on this. Save them all.

7— WITHDRAWAL: It's inevitable. It's tough. It's broken many a person's resolve before they even got going. Don't let this happen to you. You've been eating improperly for how long? Now, all of a sudden, the brakes are being hit and you simply have to push through this trying stage. It will pass! Take heart. Habits changed from unhealthy to healthy, your body tends to accommodate rather well.

8— HARD CANDY: Now, this one isn't for everybody. Only people who are able to keep hard candy in their mouth and not bite it. If you can, then your sweet tooth will be happy when you scratch the itch with something that can last for minutes instead of seconds. A slow transfusion of sugar is very strategically savvy!

9— READ and RE-READ MATERIAL: As any good student knows, nothing beats putting in the time studying. The first and 2nd time you take in new information; you're grasping to take it all in. It can be overwhelming. You'll likely miss some crucial points. You'll pick them up on repeated readings. Distraction free = more comprehension.

10— DNA DOESN'T CHEAT: No cheating. NO CHEATING! You have no say in this. You can't cheat. You either eat healthy or you don't. Your body will not co-operate with any plan or rationalization you're taking out of your excuse files. It will absorb fat, protein, carbohydrates, and calories one way. Now that you've seen the light on this, breathe a sigh of relief. It's good news. It's GREAT news, actually. The entire game of cheating can be retired!

PLAN AT 30 DAYS:

1— FLIP THE SCRIPTS: Excuses, by definition, are meant to keep you from making progress. So, avoid them. What you value, you protect. Value this endeavor and treat it like the life savior that it is. Example: Instead of the 'I can go back on a diet tomorrow' line, try 'I can eat that fattening food tomorrow'! This is a game changing mind shift. They won't quit making it, most likely. And you probably know tomorrow never really arrives. Often, the temptation will be gone.

2— TAKE A PHOTO: I did mention that there is a collage being made, right. If you've followed through with eating well, you've had a big drop in pounds. Let photos help you see the changes our eyes and head sometimes block. This is a very exciting phase. It's encouraging to see rewards quickly. Enjoy this phase because it will pass. Soon, the changes will not be so radical. Your body will begin to settle into the long term groove of a permanent lifestyle change.

3— LONG TERM PLANNING MUST BEGIN IN EARNEST: Now that you're past the initial stage and its unique challenges, it's time to plan. You won't find 'winging it' very effective. I've counseled literally thousands of people who've tried to take off weight, so my word here is backed up very reliably. I've never had anyone make it that said they 'just sort of half-heartedly tried and hoped and kinda watched it and it all worked out!' Never. Make a flexible, real world friendly attack plan and re-work it as is necessary.

4— USE CLEVER TRICKS: Who needs willpower? Willpower is very unreliable. Here are same field tested ideas to try. Eat with your opposite hand to slow you down. It works well. My habit of wolfing down food is one I still struggle with. Being left-handed, when my fork or spoon goes into my right hand, I'm suddenly unable to take more than a tiny amount and must fully concentrate or spill food all over. Plus, it's funny to watch. Put gum in your mouth to avoid nibbling. Gum is a great defense tool: It's cheap and available every-where, it keeps other foods from being mindlessly eaten. You'll find that nuts, bread, pasta, mac and cheese, sauces, meats, in fact MOST all foods suck mixed with gum. Have something to nibble on while cooking, if this is a problem for you, yes, gum works well here, too. Plus, cherry tomatoes, grapes, pickle slices all work. Now, you have something to eat while you cook that isn't going to put weight on you. This middle ground between your old ways and new ways is where most of your long term positive changes will settle.

5— TIME TO TAKE ON LEARNING ABOUT LABELS: This will be a very revealing lesson. They're very misleading. Without a degree in nutrition, here are some handy helpers. Low fat or fat free items often have high sugar content. Likewise, low sugar or sugar free items often have high fat contents. They have to get flavor or texture from somewhere. Never assume! Weasel words like reduced, in its own juice and natural fool some people. Technically, the manufacturer didn't lie. Reduced any ingredient only means it has less of some-thing than another version. It doesn't need to mean healthy at all! In its own juice can also have unhealthy things added to it. Natural, in same people's minds, automatically = healthy. Not so. Case in point, tobacco is 'natural'. In that it comes out of the ground. Kills people by the millions, too. Sugar / Salt and alternative words: use a thesau-rus for the ever changing vocabulary advertisers list things in. Many foods list sugar or salt in rather sneaky ways. You have to stay sharp to outfox the fox! <u>Serving sizes.</u> Food manufacturers are allowed to call any product as many servings as they want to give it any calorie reading they wish to dazzle you with. Ever seen a can of tuna that says it serves 4? 4 what? 4 tots? I've put a can of tuna between 2 pieces of bread, cheese and slapped mayo on it and called it a snack many times. Be mindful of a candy bar that has multiple servings to impress you with its surprisingly reasonable calorie count. When was the last time you said, 'Gee, I'd sure love 1/3 of a chocolate bar!'?

6— EXPLAIN WHAT YOU'RE DOING TO KIDS: If there are kids in your life, this is such an enormous life lesson that no child is too young to start learning. Many people overwhelm themselves with the tasks watching food is when they have kids. They're too close to see the solution that's right under their noses. Involve them! Be the judge of how much they can be involved based on their age, but don't underestimate their ability to take in more than you may think. Also, don't dismiss this life lesson for your kids if they're thin. Having thin kids has nothing to do with this. Nothing at all. They won't be growing kids forever. Knowing how to eat healthy is never not useful.

7— RE-EXAMINE MATERIAL: Yes, again. See what you pick up that was overlooked earlier. Or understand better. Training is useful, but there is no substitute for the experience you now have. It will make you see information deeper and more thoroughly.

8— RESIST DAILY WEIGHING: Some people are addicted to this. Your body cannot be rushed. Every person on the planets' body fluctuates naturally throughout the day. I've rarely met a person that obsessively, compulsively and neurotically weighs themselves that was happy. It promotes tension and stresses you. I don't even own a scale. I get weighed once a week. That is enough. I would go mad if I allowed myself to see 3 and 4 pound rises and drops that I know are occurring throughout the day. Some people disagree with me on this, but I stand by this.

9— WHO'S BEING SUPPORTIVE and WHO ISN'T: Time to evaluate if you were told, 'I'll be supportive' by anyone that has not followed though. Saying it was easy but now they've been put in the position of proving it. Who's impressed you? Who's disappointed you? For those who've gladly proven they are going to be allies in this, thank them often. They need to know how they're being helpful. Be specific about this. Let them know precisely what they're doing that you're grateful for. It makes them feel good and you're likely to get more of it. If you were surprised by the good support you received from peripheral people in your social circle, I say promote them! They need to become your new pals. Invite them to your house, to dine out, to parties... Ask your spouse. 'Do you like Tim and Elly? Good, because they're coming out with us EVERYWHERE! For those not being helpful, tell them specifically what you need from them. General statements like, 'I wish you were more supportive' may go unnoticed. I like to think the best of people. Some of us simply need guidance.

10— REMOVE FOOD FROM ONE SITUATION: You must do this in stages. It's time to begin. There are so many social events linked with food that will need unlinked. It may be a ball game without a hot dog, a movie without popcorn, buffets without dessert, card games without trays of baked goods, you decide what's first. They all have to be conquered eventually. Take on one now. You can do this!

PLAN AT 60 DAYS:

1— TAKE A PHOTO: How does it compare to your first one? You should see a noticeable difference. Smile and be happy about it. You're seeing the visible results of the hard work you're doing. This is another patch in your collage that's only going to keep looking better and better.

2— TAKE YOUR MEASUREMENTS: Add all the figures up and revel in the number. In 2 months, you've decreased your body how many inches? This process needs to only be done every other month. It's rushing it to do this more often. Left brain logic side will do a happy dance for this tangible clear evidence that you are doing so spectacularly.

3— COMPILE A 'BENEFITS SO FAR' LIST: As I've said, writing it makes it real. What's substantially better now? Acknowledge it all. Nothing is insignificant. Do you sleep better? Are you in less pain? Is there a decrease of dosage on any meds you may have been taking? Clothes? Oh, clothes that fit looser can make your day. Every belt notch, pockets that don't bulge, slacks that go on without laying down, unbuttonable things that button now - celebrate them all. Also, clothes that don't fit yet, but are improved in fit count, too. They used to go up to your hips and now you can get them up to your waist - that's progress. One day, you'll zip them. Use an article of clothing the NEXT SIZE DOWN to keep you focused. Clothes that haven't fit in years or are much smaller than you are now won't motivate in the same way. When you're tempted by food, a shirt that hasn't been worn since a few presidential elections ago can wait. But, if you have something that you can realistically be in in the next couple of months if you keep strong, well, that's relevant to your life now.

4— THROW OUT BIGGER CLOTHES: Hoarders, take note. Also, backsliding serial dieters! As clothes become too big, throw them out. Some find this tremendously difficult, but it's very necessary. Attack your resistance this way: Holding on to bigger sizes is a subliminal way of saying that you'll need them when you gain your weight back. So, backsliding is convenient, comfortable and inexpensive. You will have 90+%' paved the way for just that to happen. I want all of your momentum going in a forward direction. Put it this way, I want putting weight back on inconvenient, uncomfortable and expensive. I've had many folks return to the zone after a slip much quicker because they did that very thing. They've said that if they hadn't gotten rid of their bigger clothes, they would have continued overeating and regained much more weight. They simply don't have anything to wear and it was a choice of get back on program or re buy bigger clothes. Also, for clothes that were very expensive and worth it, have them altered. I did this with a few things: a couple jackets, a top coat and one sweater. They look great and a professional tailor made them fit like second skin. This was much cheaper and ego boosting than rebuying.

5— ASSESS DIFFICULTIES SERIOUSLY NOW: What isn't working? By now, you should be rather clear on any who, what, where, when and how's that are proving major roadblocks. My best advice, whatever you've been doing up to now, try something else. That's effective guidance I can suggest that applies to all. It's not going to resolve itself without your pro-active involvement. Be brave. Be bold. Make changes.

6— TOOLS: As needed, have I acquired the tools I must have? An insulated ice pack to bring perishable food to kids' games, a cooler for long car trips, a change of clothes for the gym in the car, foods I need for work so I don't rely on willpower against the pot lucks, vending machines and hunger pangs. Be realistic. Most of these things you need to purchase are one time investments with tremendous payoff.

7— I NEED TO DINE OUT: Perhaps you've laid low for a while. That's fine. That's smart. Learn your basics well before you test them prematurely. There is much to do and you can't take on every major challenge at once. Begin with familiar restaurants that are not at the top of your difficulty meter. Decide what you'll have before you go and stick to it. Be the first to order so you won't be swayed by suggestions. Don't even look at the menu, you don't need to. Don't go starving, ever! Some people make the mistake of stockpiling all their food for one meal out. This often backfires. All your good intentions can go right down the drain. You might eat lighter to accommodate the meal out, but take off the edge. Want to know a great tactic? Eat a piece of fruit while you're in the car on your way to the restaurant. An apple, pear, banana or whatever travels easily. It's just enough to take away ravenous feelings. If anyone asks why you're eating an apple when you're about to eat out, tell them that's exactly why, friend!

8— I CAN'T THROW OUT FOOD: Yes, you can. Any food that's tempting you - throw it out. In fact, ruin it. Put it under water, spray it with soap, pepper it inedible. Anything you need to do to make you unable to reconsider. I've had many people say they can't throw out food. Guess what, it's always fattening food. Always. I've yet to hear anyone hem or haw about being unable to throw away salad. You've thrown out mountains of veggies in your life or had a waiter take away half eaten veggies and salads. Tell the truth, you never gave it a 2nd thought. But, somehow, we pull the 'I was raised by parents that grew up in the depression' (it's been so long, that's not likely true) or 'I'll save it for work, the neighbor, whomever' when it's pasta, casseroles, cakes and the like. When was the last time you knocked on a friend's door and offered them your uneaten broccoli? Whenever you know the foods going into one of two holes, the trash can or your mouth, choose the right hole! Pretend its salad.

9— SUBTANTIAL SNACKING: A great tool of mine. No one told me this one. I came up with it. For long term satisfaction, junk doesn't cut it. Sugary, high fat, high carb, fried foods only open Pandora's box for many and leave you hungry again very soon at a high calorie count. It's unproductive. To cross over to this idea, you must unlock conventional thinking about what you eat when you eat it. This proved a game changer for me. Light frozen meals are wise mid-afternoon things to eat. Much longer lasting than chips, crackers, cookies and the last danish from the morning. There are several choices for this purpose. Or, microwave a potato. Where is it written that you can't eat a hot spud at 2PM? No place, that's where. If co-workers stare, let them. They're likely admiring your genuine efforts to improve yourself. If they say anything, tell them exactly why you're doing it. Snacking on light, meal oriented foods, it's very wise.

10— DON THE UNIFORM: Don't go to parties, restaurants or others' homes with a gloomy looking face or ta1k about how great everything looks but, alas, you can't have any. Nothing good will come of that. It'll only encourage food pushers. It's blood in the water to the sharks. You'll hear, 'don't be a drag', 'you've been so good, you deserve it' or this classic, 'It's just one night'. Shine it on in a low key manor and you'll invite less pushing and stress. This doesn't come naturally at first. You have to don the uniform of this person before it becomes unforced. Even if you're not feeling anywhere near as confident inside, don't let on. To be a warrior, you need the armor for protection. There's no fault in this, it's very wise. With time, you'll become more accustomed to the fit.

PLAN AT 90 DAYS:

1—TAKE A PHOTO: You're dressing differently to accentuate and profess your accomplishments now. If you're clinging to clothes that're much too big for you still, examine why. Are you hiding? Calling it comfort when they're other reasons? There's no need. The hatchling is emerging from the shell. It's a new world, don't be afraid!

2— PUSH PAST LULLS: It isn't new anymore. Avoid the panic that can strike at this point. What panic? It really WILL be necessary to monitor my eating forever to keep this weight loss going - gasp! The thrill is gone, then? No, the 'new car' smell is. Ultimately, the novelty phase must wear off. You're seeing the view on a level playing field now. Just take another step ahead.

3— WHAT HABITS FEEL UNFORCED: Now is the perfect time to stretch as far as you can to pat yourself on the back. When all of this is new, it's all forethought, time, repetition, caution, calculations, verifying, forcing you to get back up on the horse. The victories come in stages, not as one plans. See what you're doing that's no longer quite a struggle. See what you're doing that feels entirely natural now. Use this encouragement to nurture confidence and know that soon, all areas will improve.

4— KEEP DINING OUT: Find the easier places. You need doable dishes all the places you'll dine. By all means, ask, ask, ASK. Ask for what? Ask for absolutely anything you need. Restaurants will do just about anything you ask that's within their kitchens' power. Menus are simply a first draft. Don't see any platter that fits what you're after. Ask the server to add this, subtract that, substitute helpful items for tempting things, don't have things on the table that you don't intend to eat. The willpower it takes to resist is a waste of energy. It takes practice and some trial and error. Don't forget, the server makes their money off your tips, it's in their interest that you're happy.

5— CONSULT OLD FOOD RECORDS, THEY'RE GOLD: Have you seen the wisdom of this? Have you benefitted by using them? They're your story and will ease struggles in a tried and very personal way that no one can compose for you. They're also time savers. If you took the time to find dishes that worked well, save them so that later on you can take the info to reuse. If you're in a more troublesome place, take an entire week as a redo. You can surrender your will one week. Respect the success it brought you not too long ago.

6— FOOD GOES BAD: Who knew! Perhaps you've noticed that as you drop food consumption down to more civil levels that your old quantities you bought are not disappearing as quickly. Maybe some foods have gone stale in the process. This particular phenomenon came later in life to me. I'd heard of food going bad, but hadn't experienced it firsthand. Items like chip clips, Tupperware, foil, cling wrap, zip lock baggies, vacuum sealers and what not were unneeded in my life. They presume you're not going to eat all you make or buy. This is Chinese talking to a Greek here. A failure to communicate if there ever was! Now, I've seen the light. Bread molds after a certain time. Chips get stale. Ice collects on frozen items. Meat rots. Cheese turns other colors. Even ketchup goes all watery-like. All concepts you have to see to believe. I'm a late bloomer. Shop with common sense.

7— While common sense is being discussed, I believe that's an inaccurate pairing of words. Common sense is not common. I wish it was. It's rather uncommon, in my life's experience, particularly with food. Here's a great example: You don't have to love everything you eat; you have to LIKE it. This colossal shift was another game changer for me. A massive earthquake game changer, really. My love for food was so all encompassing that love was too weak a word for it. What's beyond love? Double love? Deluxe love? Mega love? Words fail me. I talk for a living, words rarely fail me so this is a big statement in and of itself. You don't have to love every single thing you eat; you have to like it. Has it sunk in any? When it does, you may find your mind open to all sorts of possible meal, snack, cooking and dining out options that would not have been welcomed in before. Now, the waters are less rapid and the sailing coasts smoother. Why? Because I've allowed it! Liking what you eat is very underrated. You are calm, satisfied and willing to come to the challenge table another day when you like what's being offered. Love factors in - of course it does. But it doesn't have a lockdown on your choices, either. For example, I don't love lettuce, pears, light bread, fat free yogurt, turkey, sugar tree popsicles, powdered cream or Whopper juniors. I like them enough, though. I love being thin and healthy. Those foods contribute to my higher achievement and thus merit my great respect. Love what you like!

8— SEE THE WOLF UNDER THE SHEEPSKIN: You're not a yearling now. Wise up. Resist the 'I need a break' cliché. You've allowed the rot to set in too many times in the past with this one, haven't you? What's your success history with this? Pretty abysmal, is it? Well, come sit next to me because I understand you. You're like me, normal. When I test this, I fall down flat on my face every time. Truth be told, I DON'T need a break when I say this. Neither do you. We both know this. What I need is a break from taking breaks! Hear that noise? It was another smart bomb exploding in your mind.

9— DO SOMETHING THAT SCARES YOU A BIT: You may see the ever annoying life stream that you seem to benefit greatly from this. Some of us, when we get good advice, hear it, heed it and live better. How simple. Others seem perpetually in need of testing it and taking lumps in the process. Which side do you fall on? Don't self-criticize this too much. But, yes, keep on. You don't need to select #1 on your list at first, maybe #5. It's conquerable and sets an 'achiever's mind set' in you. That'll help you tackle more trying things better. Realistic preparations and expectations are building blocks people have climbed mountains upon.

10— FORWARD ROWING ONLY: Your reasons for beginning this may be solved or not factor into your day to day life now. Is that bad? No, it's not, but it can pose long term problems you didn't count on that you are at the stage to fall from. What do I mean? Hear me out. I have watched many, many people lose around 50% of their weight and the fire seems unexplainably at 50% with it. How do get the pilot light back on more reliably? Build, stoke and keep watch in constantly forward focused ways. Your initial game plan has served you well, but needs rearranging or you risk idling, stalling, frustration and backsliding. Goals more towards your future and less about your past are the new rocket fuel.

PLAN AT 365 DAYS:

1— TAKE A PHOTO: Collage at a year. Put them together and take the transformation in. What do you want to do with it? Frame it, keep it to yourself? Time goes quickly. Remember thinking this would take so long? Look, just look at you now. The slim you is the 'real' you, even if you're meeting for the first time. Greet 'real you' warmly. 'Real you' has been very patient waiting for this day.

2— TAKE MEASUREMENTS: The right side of the brain just got an overflow fix. Now, douse the left side with impressive stats like your 1 year measurements. Aren't you glad you documented the first ones? There wouldn't be this glorious info now if you hadn't. Well done, you!

3— ALL BIG CLOTHES ARE GONE: This should have happened. If not, celebrate your day 365 milestone by making good on this. However, keep one thing. The biggest thing you ever had to buy. The one that crushed you you'd eaten your way up to. This single reminder of what you could return to if you get influenced by media, friends, your old ways or new situations you couldn't have forecasted. A reminder that a cure isn't on the map to be discovered, my bridge to fitting back into it has been burned.

4— SCHEDULED MILESTONES: You know the birthdays, anniversaries, baptisms, national holidays, personal ones are coming. How did I manage? They will all repeat. How to celebrate without food is a learned behavior. Continue to view your life differently.

5— PASS IT ONTO KIDS: This is for any children in your life. They look to you to guide them. As tough as you found this undertaking, you have a golden opportunity to break the cycle. When you don't have celebrations centered around food with kids, it's their normal. They won't grow up with the baggage to unlearn. It's a very loving gift to pass on. There is a great commercial for a certain cookie mix that's shown at Christmas. The adult and kid are making a small amount of cookies, one gingerbread man per kid that they customize with icing, sprinkles and such. But the emphasis is on the loving connection between them. The food is secondary. The warm fuzzy holiday sweet moment will still happen if you bake one dozen as it might with multiple dozens. At least as far as the child is concerned.

6— UNEXPECTED CHALLENGES: Life has many of them: weddings, sicknesses, job changes, deaths, moving, injuries and more. Did you remain steadfast? What could you have done to improve in the future? If you are only able to reign in your eating when it's easy, then you can't reign in your eating. In stress, what will overeating do? Distract you, then make what was stressing you in the first place even worse. Also, you've reintroduced potential binge foods into your system and added guilt, indigestion, needs to put wrappers under trash cans, lie about forgetting a certain kind of hair conditioner so you need to run to the store to get more.... wow, you'd gotten used to being done with this game and now look at this? When your ducks are any way except in a row, and you still know you are not going to overeat over it, then you're coping in the most productive way possible. You're a pro.

7— COOK1NG and DINING OUT SHOULD BE EASY NOW: Is that possible? Yes, it is. I'm going to go bold here. Nothing's too tough that it can't be surmounted. Men have walked on the moon, remember? Can I order food in a restaurant? Can I cook a new way? Yes! I have a list of over 30 places I have eaten in the last 2 years with meals I could eat and not feel a twinge of worry over. This only happened the way it does for all of us —I put in the time. I don't have tempting foods in my house because I'm not cured. I know how to use seasoning, lean meats, wisely chosen frozen items and know how to grill, bake, broil and microwave with aplomb! As for eating out, they don't TELL you what to order, do they? It's only a problem if you go starving (an apple before I go is 2nd nature now) or unprepared (with time, you never need to be). When you hear the old excuses from others, you may find it tough to pipe down about how untrue they are. Just look good, smile calmly and those with ears, minds and hearts open will ask. And hear.

8— HOW HAVE I CHANGED MY LIFESTYLE: Hobbies that are physical (live the dreams - sail, swing dance, Zumba, bike ride, run marathons, rock climb, fly kites, ride a balloon, anything I only watched and dreamt of are now reality), job changes (they require confidence, research and learning new skills - do I wish to break out?), non-toxic friendships (I no longer have some people in my life because they don't need to be. Others proved worthy and are cherished. I'm not sad about the others. I don't dwell on them), health improvements (it feels amazing to live without heart palpitations, belabored breathing, insulin injections, asthma inhalers, tubes of muscle ache ointments, dental trouble, skin trouble, heartburn, gas, excessive sweating and on and on with the laundry list of what can go wrong when you live too long too overweight. With a dose of sanity, I see that no food is worth living like that for), self-esteem (either I knew it was in the gutter and I accepted it or I didn't think about it at all for risk of feeling miserable). I have a life now. I have MY life now. I will do the work to remain this person.

9— REMEMBER CONSEQUENCES: Bad times can bring up food cravings. Good times can bring up food cravings. Dull times can bring up food cravings. Well, what times does that leave? When are you not feeling good, neutral or bad? When you're asleep? No one waved a magic wand over you to grant you what you now have. It was work. Still, you can't simply un-know what you know. Yes, there was fun in glutting out from Thanksgiving to New Years' and not caring. Knowing you'd return from vacations not fitting into anything that fit when you packed. Staying in the shadow of excuses everyone accepted and ate to distraction. There are times I wistfully look back and wish I could "just let go". But, I know I cannot. I am addicted to overeating and like an alcoholic can't "just let go" on a cruise with a promise to get back on the wagon when I'm back on land. Many try and many relapse via that thinking. The one and only true useful thing about looking back to your past is to counterattack any strong desires to step into bear traps. Focus on how your life is better. I don't even give myself a gluttony pass on my birthday. I've been pushed to many times. While my willpower goes up and down like all of us, I remember the damage and do what I need to. My birthday is celebrated with a small cake with one candle. Then I don't resist more cake and I fit in what I wore to my own party. Never forget how miserable you were before. It's a power source when you have to say, "No, thank you" to tempting food. You need to *sound* like you mean it and you *need* to mean it.

10— YOU DON'T CATCH OBESITV: In our ever more non responsibility taking world, it seems we're coming around to treating obesity like a disease or condition you did nothing to bring on, such as a common cold. No, it's deliberate. You ate what you ate and put every pound on one at a time. This being said, this is also the well your recovery feeds from. It's entirely in your own power to never be overweight again. Your ethnicity, environment, economic status and all other personal exteriors contribute to the level of difficulty, but don't dictate your destiny. Know this and you're thin forevermore.

PROLOGUE - WHY DO WE OVER CONSUME:

This was the toughest section to write. Its messages are hard facts for many. By many, I mean millions. I cannot offer more precise quantifications. I'm just one of the fortunate ones who detached from the freight train of self-destructive over consumption. With that, my vantage point changed. Do you understand? If not, I mean a healthy dose of sanity took over and my perspective shifted with it. My, oh, my - how did I live like I did for so many years? My need to eat was at optimum level at least 90% of the time and no amount ever quenched it. It nearly killed me. It kills many. Insurance companies are feeling the strain overweight client's claims are costing. It truly is an epidemic.

Various proposals are analyzed. This is my attempt to shake you up and into a willingness to see your whole existence differently. Observe yourself with a 3rd person vantage point and it all may sink in more effectively. Next, we annihilate complacency, passivity and denial.

Sounds serious – It is. A re-reading of this section while making revisions overwhelmed me. It was as though I was coming to it for the first time. That's a good litmus test to its validity and power. Please, let it sink in and commit to being a member of the 'exception to the rule clan. One by one, we can add to its force and eventually reclaim ourselves and redirect the next generation.

Is it too late? I don't think so. I'll never give up. We can still do this, people! If you're still alive, it's not too late. If you feel the reasons we over consume that are discussed here have overtaken you - the anti-venom is here, also.

WHY DO WE OVER-CONSUME - 10 THEORIES:

Before I begin, let me be clear about what is here, a collection of theories. Theories, by definition, are rational contemplations. However, I feel it important that I first give my credentials regarding this. Without them, this chapter would not be of any substance. Three credible reasons to hear me out.

One - Personal experience. I was an overweight child, an overweight teen and everything from a thin to chubby to overweight to morbidly obese adult. I've lived a life where overconsumption of food has never been far from the core. No other source was needed to compile any of this. They're all byproducts of living in the whirlpool of over consuming's aftereffects. I have lived many of these and battled them.

Two - Field tested. In my over 16 years of working with the public regarding weight loss, I have been able to do much more than observe. I've personally dealt with thousands upon thousands of men, women and minors from all walks of life and have been privy to insights I would not have had access to any other way. These theories require much time, repetition and study to come to any reliable conclusions. Internet polls were not consulted for their opinions. Years have been spent taking all data discussed.

Three – Fact check. There is easily verifiable proof you can research on your own to comply with facts shared here. Don't agree with something, find out what's true.

1— PHYSICAL PLEASURE: I begin with the easiest culprit. Many foods just taste so good. What keeps you distracted? Pizza, chips, ice cream, hamburgers, cookies, fried chicken, bread and butter, nuts, chocolate bars, bacon, doughnuts, ranch dressing, French fries, beer, crackers, burritos.... all of this and more? Of course! While eating, it's a sensation like no other. Your body literally needs it. Unlike vices your body doesn't need and can, frankly, do perfectly fine without, food rides the dangerous middle ground. I'm alternatively giving my body what it needs and abusing it to such excess with my poor choices. I've turned a biological need into a staggering problem. Like intentionally breathing in polluted air, I slowly contaminate myself. Who in their right mind does that? Well, no one in their right mind! The lure of food can overtake your judgment. Food is not only delicious and satisfying, but in most places, it's easily gotten, costs range from very expensive to dirt cheap, completely legal and requires no involvement from anyone else. This = a perfect storm for becoming obese. Many poisons please the senses.

2— RESTAURANTS: To remain competitive, the shift in the last 30 years has been to ever upsize portions when dining out. Where is this going to end? I have had members in the restaurant business confirm what I already knew was true. The standard size china was increased in the 80s across the US. I have watched while portions that would have been put in the middle of a table for a family to pick from are put in front of individuals. If a restaurant opened today and served what would have been adequate amounts in 1978, they'd be out of business in a flash. In this land of milk and honey we're become dwellers in a land of milk shakes and honeybuns. It isn't pretty. It also doesn't seem to be enough. Forget 30 and 40 years ago, I've seen portions jump up noticeably since the mid to late 1990s even further. You can only blame the pusher of a substance to a certain extent. They are fulfilling a need. If they put out full troths of food and no one bought it, they'd change strategies. They only want to make money. Some animals don't know when to stop. They're natural instincts are to glut on any food until it's all gone or they are literally incapable of taking in anymore. Are we among those animals?

3— STIGMA IS DROPPED: A very double edged sword. True story: I was in line at a famous sandwich store and the guy in front of me was having difficulty with the young lady behind the counter regarding his order. Each item he asked for was being sprinkled on and he was gruffly saying, 'more than that' with obvious edge in his voice. When he went away, the young lady went on a break and the manager took my order. I mentioned what had just happened. He sighed and explained, the young lady was a college exchange student from France and they were having problems with her. She didn't understand how Americans eat and he was trying to tell her to be more generous. i.e.: You don't sensibly glaze mayo on sandwiches here, you glob it. His very words: "This is America, we eat like pigs. Pile it on." He said she was always going on about how much we eat and how disgusting we are. A patriotic man like me can only take offence to a certain point. Through her eyes, it's probably a very common reaction.

To put it another way, I was one of about 4 or 5 truly overweight kids in my elementary school. We were all teased a lot. Not good times. Now, it's less uncommon to be overweight as a kid, so they don't stand out as much. Some may not endure the level of teasing we had.

That's a good thing, definitely. No child should be picked on. But there is an unhappy side to this no one can deny. Kids are heavier than ever. Many teachers have been among my students and agree. They've watched the kids get bigger and bigger as the years pass. It's as though there was a lens focusing in on a class photo making it larger and larger. Ultimate irony - in my youth, if I misbehaved, I could be threatened with being told if I didn't toe the line, I would not be allowed to go outside. This threat worked. That got me acting right. Staying inside all weekend or after school? UGH. Now, parents tell me the threat they level over kids as potential punishment is that they MUST go outside. With no mobile devices, they see the fear in their small faces.

4— CULTURE COP OUT: Let's drop this one, ok? I've heard every nation on the planet (well, no one's mentioned Malta to my face yet, but I'm sure it's coming) blamed for why people are overweight. "You don't understand, I'm ish, we eat." My, oh, my, as opposed to where? Where do they NOT eat? These lucky stiffs in land exist on oxygen and osmosis and don't eat food. Really? Bring it closer to home, if you prefer. I've had many states and U.S. cities blamed as well. "I'm from the Midwest, the South, New Orleans, San Francisco, Chicago, New York, the country side, Miami, Texas…we eat." If you expect cart blanche on having to correct yourself via your land of upbringing I will not oblige. I was raised in a Greek and Middle Eastern family that was very food oriented. In Las Vegas, buffets abound. I could stay huge until my earlier-than-it- had-to-be death if I simply stood still on that. Pacific Islanders have high percentages of overweight. Japanese do not. There is less obesity in the Pacific Northwest in America. But until you tell me there is tangible evidence EVERVONE of a region or ethnicity is obese and it's scientifically verified that it's in their DNA, I won't accept this as justification. Poor eating habits permeate everyplace. Good ones can be planted and grown, too.

Culture is a cop out. Some traditions need to endure, some need to be altered and some need to end.

5— FEAR OF SUCCESS: Strange thing to say to some. Yes, there are people who seem afraid of success. Over-consuming and remaining overweight can be manifestations of this. With success in weight loss, there are expectations. While I do not have a fear of success, I did have a somewhat similar unpleasant side effect of losing weight in 1977 discussed in my own story. At 275+#, my non-dating could be written off. As a thin guy, my being gay was brought to the forefront and I did not like it. Lots of overweight people do complain a lot, but then don't take steps to change it. I've broached this in meetings and seen squirming members that are being prodded where they didn't like. If I'm single, it's because I'm so big and men (or women) are so superficial they can't see the 'real inner me' and so they aren't worth dating. Well, it sounds nice, but doesn't tackle the deeper issue. If you lose weight, you'll be expected to dress up, go out and compete to get a man or woman. What's the reason you're single now? Maybe your personality isn't appealing underneath all the extra pounds. In this same vein, if you have a lousy job and you're overweight, it's the unfair stigma against you that's holding you back and your boss is unfair promoting that less qualified but thinner guy over you. Maybe so, there is DEFINITELY a stigma unfairly held against overweight people. Life isn't fair, is it? If you lose your weight, now why don't you have a better job? You'll be expected to dress up, compose an impressive resume, get out, pound the pavement, sell yourself, shine on interviews and make a better career for yourself. Success can bring responsibility and higher expectations. It's enough for some to stay comfortably, miserably uncomfortable and lament what could have been.

6— HIDING: The extra size is a literal, physical barrier used as a personal weapon by choice. It keeps people away. They can't touch you, hug you or get dose. Some people are put off emotionally by obese people and stay away for that reason, too.

I've watched and participated in seminars where victims of rape and childhood molestation say they became obese as a defense reflex. Intentionally becoming unattractive sexually and not be hurt again. Burying all the horrific memories and fears under crippling layers of extra pounds may seem like the safest thing to do in a wounded state of mind. Too often, the catastrophic consequences don't begin to be seen as needed to be dealt with until they've eaten themselves into a truly dangerous situation.

7— HOSTILITY: Internally directed anger = body abuse in many. Some choose cutting, some abuse drugs, some become promiscuous; others select overeating as their self-destruction. While it can be obvious when a person is close to rock bottom, before it reaches that point, it's often covered up. A frequent defense can be donning an 'I don't care' type of armor. Underneath is a broiling hostility you'd scald yourself with if touched. You aren't safe, sane and certainly not healthy. You must redirect anger. This factored into a couple of profiles. If you come from a family of overweight people, it's alright. No, it isn't. If you can live too calmly and peacefully with your extra weight, it's very unlikely you'll have the fire to change it. Feel the anger. Be entirely ticked off with yourself and focus it into the direction of change. Others will pick up on this, as well. Instead of denying anger and playing a role you're insincerely delivering and likely not fooling anyone with anyway - take yourself in hand and get the weight off. Positive atmospheres will come to you. Friends will accept and admire you or know not to say anything because you're too strong to be influenced. Negative people, you've learned to turn off the negative noise. This brings peace.

8— IT'S BEEN MADE TOO COMFORTABLE: Untucked tops, elastic waistbands, stretch pants, jogging suits as casual daywear, pajamas as acceptable public attire, too. A generation ago, this would have been ridiculous. How many of you dress for work in a way your parents would have been sent home for if they'd shown up like that? The option wasn't on the table. I'll never forget the first time I had a certain mother and daughter join my class. I took a double shot at them. Only after repeated glances did I really believe my eyes - they were wearing pajamas in public. I was so put off. How trashy they seemed. Years pass, now it doesn't even turn my head in the grocery store. Truthfully, WE WANT DENIAL. Clothing labels have changed to assist in this. Don't forget, I am a buyer of plus sized clothing from many years back. My word is reliable here. As we became more and more overweight, companies realized they would lose sales if their customers were unhappy with reminders of their size. Seemingly overnight, there were no more humiliating XXL, XXXL, XXXXLs and so on. Labels became 1X, 2X, 3X, 4X. You're still the same size, but it stung less. We bought into it quickly. For ladies' clothes came a new word for bigger sizes: women's. We all know the 'woman's section' of a department store is where the larger sizes are. What does 'woman' mean here - bigger, wider and stretchier. I recall when the places you bought those clothes were called "Big men's" and "Big woman's" shops. Can you imagine such an appallingly politically incorrect store opening today named that? They'd be protested out of business in a month.

No, no, no. Businesses exist to make money, so they do whatever they need to do to get yours. Happily, they'll help delude you. Like restaurants had to get bigger plates for the general public, standard clothing sizes have gotten bigger patterns and redefined the meaning of labels. Want proof of this: go on any vintage website or EBay and read descriptions of the sizing. They all explain it somewhat the same. If it's decades old, you can't gage your size by the label of what you're bidding on. A good overall monitor - Men's shirts: Today's S = 70s M. Today's M = 70s L. Today's L = 70s XL. Today's XL = 70s big man's store. Women's patterns: Today's 6 = 70s 8. Today's 10 = 70s 12. Today's 14 = 70s 16. Today's 18 = 70s big woman's store. I can't even describe the recalculations kids' clothes have gone through. Sad. Sad. Sad.

9— MOB MENTALITY: Scary and dangerous. Case in point: If a law exists and no one obeys it, it becomes unenforceable. You can't ticket the entire city if a stop sign keeps continually being driven through. More people are followers than leaders. They simply do what the majority of people around them do. Rocking the boat just isn't in their mind skill set or nature. Over consuming food and living overweight is so common now that it's claiming many more citizens via mob mentality. We're effectively damaging beyond what can even projected for our future if this doesn't stop. I'm very worried about this one.

10— ACCEPTANCE: Possibly the worst of all. I saved it for last. A life passively lived in acceptance of your state. Being overweight early brings on this incorrect mind view sooner and the damage worsens. As years go by, the extra weight, the burden your bear, the cumbersome nature of it, the diminished energy level, the low self-esteem, the illnesses you must expect, the pain you feel, the unimpressive appearance you ignore, the passing on of all of this to your children, the lack of ambition or belief you're meant to be anything other than what you are intertwine and you create a ball and chin. You take this ball and chain from the welding factory and latch it on. Then you drag it through your existence.

You can't go through days, weeks and years actively hating yourself. It just isn't productive. You ignore it. After time, the ball and chain becomes less noticed. It becomes a part of you. You don't dwell on the fact that it's dragging you down constantly. Please, wake up, see the ball and chain, SEE IT for what it is: removable. Yes, you ate in on, but the glorious truth is that you can eat it off, too. Recovery comes to those get mad, look within, reach out, turn the key and detach the ball and chin. Then, you're free forevermore.

PROLOGUE RECIPES:

Imagine being a perfectionist who can't get anything right, or a disorganized person suffering from OCD or a vet allergic to dogs? This section will not be what you expect. I'm using the word recipe loosely. I don't believe in assuming. But, here it may be valid for you, the reader, to make the conclusion you're about to get step-by-step instructions on preparing dishes and meals. The assumption is ½ right.

There will be a few. But more so, I'm dealing with the extraneous parts of kitchen duty. This is not meant to mislead or cheat you out of any useful knowledge. I'm not withholding. On the contrary, I don't hold much back as a general rule. It's simply that I know very little about traditional cooking. What I do know is temperature changes, spicing, portion distortion, viewing foods for their long term hunger management and keeping kitchens free of what needs to be absent. Then, you're not living in a mine field.

I am food obsessed and I don't like cooking. I've never learned much beyond the most basic and simple things to throw together. My eating habits were sated by looking outwards. Now, my utter lack of respect for pre-set rules has served me well as I constructed my own version of 'standard eating' out of blocks and mud pies. Yet, it's kept me thin for many years. Keep that in the front of your mind. It can work for you, too.

No, I don't have the home people go to for the parties where all the delicious food is. I leave that role for others. What I get is invited to many other folk's homes and their parties. I earn my keep by being a lively guest with gifts for my hosts, joining in whatever fun they're trying to get the overstuffed fuddy duddies to do (karaoke? - ok, charades? —yes, walk in the park? - no trouble, backyard volleyball? - fun, dancing? - born to boogie, just about anything!). Leave the food to the restaurateur. I can be the raconteur. Keep being open to change and bon appétit!

X485'S RECIPES AND COOKING TIPS:

As way of an intro here, let me confess: I hate cooking. I don't cook when it can be avoided. I think I didn't have kids because of the 20-year cooking obligation. Is it mysterious considering my life- long food obsession that I hate cooking? Well, I'm not sure. I love clothes and I don't like to sew, either. Moral: a fondness for consuming something isn't automatically connected to any desire to create it. So, there.

In my lifetime, I've seen a shift in this area. The advancement of quality frozen foods (healthy or otherwise) has transformed US cooking. Microwave preparation has advanced to allow finer tasting foods in them. The growing number of single adults that don't want or need to cook meals for a family has contributed to this, as well. As a cooking hater, I feel I'm exactly in the right place at the right time. You don't have to know how to cook anymore. It's a choice. In previous generations, it was a life skill. Adults needed to know how to cook, especially women. Now, it's an option. Learn to cook if it interests you or...just go out.... or the microwave, crock pot and toaster oven are all you need to remain blissfully, unapologetically uninvolved in food preparation.

So, why an Earth is there an X485's recipes and cooking tips section to this book? What do I have of any merit to offer? Well, there is the matter of losing 300# and keeping it off for over 16 years as a pre qualifier for my credentials on food, in general. More to the point, I am often asked how I've managed to do what I've done and NOT cook. So, I share my best secrets in my desire to help all those suffering. Suffering from what, you may wonder? Traditions that keep one tied to unhealthy cooking and obligations interfering with lightening your food. Inexperience at scaling back food quantities in general is a huge struggle for many. They just need a few hints to disengage from the kitchen.

Few of these offerings are actual recipes, in any way. The rest are strategies to switch your daily routines towards a more weight loss consistent direction.

1— VEGGIE SOUP IN A TROTH: Sound tasty? It's my life line. What I so classily call a 'troth' is a mold for baking bread. Baking and I broke up long ago. But, I use the baking items as much as if we hadn't. I make huge veggie soups in them at least 3 times a week for dinner, sometimes, more than that. A typical one is 1 can diced tomatoes, 1 can carrots, 1 can green beans, 1 can corn, 1 can mushrooms, onions (fresh or dehydrated) and pepper, pour in V-8, stir and microwave for 8 minutes. Stir it up so it's all well mixed. Microwave the 90 second white rice. Throw it in and good eating! I owe my maintenance to this dish. If you want more heat, hot sauce does the job. When I visit family, I have to go to the grocery store to stock up on the canned veggies to make this. It's indispensable. It's filling to the point of struggling to finish it. It's healthy, hot, tasty and easy to make. You can alter the menu for other veggies, of course: peppers, broccoli, eggplant...whatever veggie you can fit in the troth - go for it. The rice gives it just the right amount of carbohydrate kick to allow it to be called a meal. Oh, and feel free to add meat or beans. I've been hungrier than usual some nights and kicked up its oomph with protein. There's no way to do this wrong, really.

To convince you to buy into the veggie troth more, let me tell you some more of its perks beyond the so-helpful-it's-insane for your diet ones. NEXT TO NO CLEAN UP: Being lazy in the kitchen has worked to my advantage. No cutting board, knives or multiple pots or pans or rice cookers to bother with when you're tipping over from troth consumption. Cans go right into the trash, yes, they do. An electric can opener is a must, too! PATH TO DESSERT: My sweet tooth is relentless.

If yours is, too, then the veggie troth gets 'em in! With so few calories to worry about, it's been my saving grace dinner if lunch was overboard (planned or unplanned, it still works!) or if my need for sugar must be met. What more needs to be said?

2— HUGE SALADS: Yes, I grant you, salads are the par-for-the-course item on diets, yet they don't have to be dull. I admit, I'm lucky here, in that I love veggies. They're not punishment. Even in my heaviest days, salads and veggies were welcome parts of my meals. So, when I decided fattening food and I needed to see other people, salad was the friend waiting patiently in the wings. I leaned on them from the get go and still do. I use them to manage hunger. Similar to the veggie troth, I make them BIG. My personal salads are often in what I believe is meant to be a family salad bowl. No worries when you live alone of anyone judging you. Although, I've eaten this in front of others many times, too. Here is a basic breakdown. PRECUT BAGS OF LETTUCE: Being lazy in the kitchen pays off, again! How happy am I that you don't even have to chop up heads of lettuce anymore! The bag options are many. Which mix this time? They have many sealing options but they don't apply to me since I intend to not seal them. But, if you're looking to use only 1/2 of one, by all means, read the labels for what works best for you. CHERRY TOMATOES: You don't even have to cut these, are you kidding me? I know they're not the best tasting ones, but they're ready to eat size, so they're in. ONIONS: I'm addicted. So much so that I have chopped them in the old school way to get them in. For me, that's saying a lot. Being lazy in the kitchen lead me to a mini food processer to eliminate this task. My first time washing it, I didn't realize quite how sharp the blades are, picked it up clumsily and cut myself pretty badly. Walking upstairs to the bathroom with blood coming out alarmingly from my right hand I took this as a sign from God that cooking is evil and to be avoided. So, I found pre-cut onions and never looked back. How had I missed them? Man! SCALLIONS and CUCUMBERS: Sigh, I must peel and cut these to this day. It's not my favorite thing, but I must make the sacrifice if I'm to have salads with proper variety. So, I endure the 5 minutes of agony to do this for myself. Mix items with any variety of vinegars, oils and spices that suits your palate. CRACKERS: Crumble a few on top for crunch and fridge uncovered to get it good and cold. Feel free to supplement them with proteins as desired like in the troth recipe. Beans, cold meat, hot meat, starchy veggies like corn can all consider themselves invited to the party. Finish the barrel full!

Good reader, how can I convince you of the wisdom of this? It gets you thin. It keeps you thin. Your hunger is managed and that's invaluable. Hot or cold, troth or barrel, veggies are your ally in this.

3— HOT / COLD SWITCH-ER-OO: A very effective way to bring interest into your eating is to look at foods in the opposite temperature than is commonly used to serve them. Not everything works here, but many DO! I've doubled my ways to enjoy healthy and filling foods by turning up the heat (or, to be real, punching the microwave longer) or cooling off many things. Here are some examples.

USUALLY SERVED HOT, BUT ARE GREAT COLD - **beans** (black, red, white, kidney, black eyed peas, pinto, all beans work well), **beef** (it gets less press than cold meats of other varieties, now you can put in on salads, yea!), **soup** (a gourmet concept for a few styles only? No way. Cold soups are great. Open your mind and open wide), **corn** (less popular, this yellow delight is passed up too often if it's not hot), **spaghetti** (granted, it's not light, but if you've prepared it sensibly and the portion is reasonable, last night's Italian doggie bag treat is great right out of the fridge), **grapes** (not usually served hot, I know. But try them frozen, it's amazing). What are some other foods you've found a temp twist on from hot to cold? Let me know and I might try them!

USUALLY SERVED COLD, BUT ARE GREAT HOT - **pudding** (oh, MAN, the best! Trust me on this), **fruit** (some of you are aware of this, but I'll bet you don't do it enough. Heated fruit ROCKS! Grilled, micro waved, baked or otherwise, apples, pineapples, peaches, pears, plums…I could go on and on), **tuna** (another diet perennial that I find MUCH tastier hot than cold. It isn't just for casseroles, either. Heated tuna works with many dishes), **milk** (never a favorite beverage of mine, unless it's heated and flavored. Then, bring it on!), **nuts** (the Christmas song got this right. They're not only delicious, but too hot to wolf down). What are some other foods you've found a temp twist on from cold to hot? Let me know and I might try them!

4— TIME RESTRICTIONS RELEASED - A complete game changer for food. When I let go of any restrictions on what I ate when I ate, it was a piñata exploding with possibilities. Suddenly, I was able to eat, keep satisfied and diet mentality went goodbye if I saw foods differently: as in on no schedule. I cannot overstate how effective this is. Where is it written, it's written no place, that you can't microwave a light meal at 2:30pm at work, or at 10:50am? When I got this in my head, I began popping bags of popcorn while the tray of bagels came around. Baked potatoes as snacks, YES! The smell would attract comments such as, 'You're eating a potato at so and so time?' Yes, I was and I couldn't have felt smarter when I was driving past all the fast food drive through places that I'd made my regular stops on the way home. I wasn't just passing them by via willpower, I wasn't hungry! Tuna fish sandwiches for breakfast - great! Two slices of grilled roast beef with oil at 10 when others were having pastry - yes, thank you. Oatmeal, toast and fruit for dinner— light and delightful! Heartier lunches seemed to be worked off for the energy and calories better than the normal sit in front of the tv or computer most of us do after dinner. Therefore, if there was going to be a choice to indulge in red meat, pasta or dessert, most times it was at lunch. Steamable sides were heated and eaten at mid-afternoon because I could see them as not stuck as side dishes. Salads as late night snacks to gnaw on - aces! These are only habits you were brought up with, they have no bearing on the way you live now. I felt like I'd unlocked a secret that could change my very future when I glommed onto this. You know what, it did.

5— OILS, SPICES, VINEGARS and CONDIMENT CONTROL: I love options. Give me choices and I'm happy. Want to get on my bad side where food is concerned: tell me there's a set menu. I despise them. Tell me the chef likes to prepare it this way. Well, this customer likes to **EAT** it **THIS** way. Since you're saying 'we need to see other people' to many foods and embracing healthier ones you need to know how to make them engaging. Oils, spices and vinegars have come light years in the last decade in choice and easy availability. They have their own sections of the markets where there used to be much fewer choices. Learn what they all taste like, what they mix well with and use them generously. We all know about olive oil, red and white standard vinegar, salt, pepper, cinnamon, butter, ketchup, mustard and mayo. There are oodles and zillions more of all of these to make your meals come alive and taste many different ways. Begin in the discount stores and buy the smallest container of anything you're unfamiliar with so you're not stuck with too much if you don't like it. I'm sure most oils, vinegars, spices and condiments you'd taste and say, 'Oh, I know that, it's on_____.' Well, good for you for taking step 1. Now, put them in soups, salads, sides, eggs, ground beef, salsas, pasta sauces, all meats .... learn to experiment and have a full cabinet of them all and you'll feel like a scientist in a laboratory making creations that'll zap boredom out of any low fat - calorie thing you eat. i.e.: salsa on salads - yummy, cumin in soup - yes. Oils go virtually anyplace butter can go (what did you think was glistening on grilled cheese sandwiches or garlic bread, anyway?). Go for it!

6— OPEN MINDED-NESS WITH COOKBOOKS - We've all been guilty of this one. How many potentially tasty recipes have you dismissed out of magazines, cookbooks or online because you looked at a single ingredient? Mistake! Like when people look at homes, it's the bones of the thing you need to focus on. When buyers talk about the paint or light fixtures, it must drive realtors crazy trying to stifle groans of 'It's easily fixable. Look at the structure of the place, you ninny!' Likewise, if a dish says 'spicy this or that' and you say, 'Oh, my husband doesn't like spicy food' and you turn the page, turn back. Taking out the heat is the easiest thing in the world to do. It may, otherwise, have been an enjoyable dish. Stews, soups, casseroles, omelets, salads and many recipes can have a meat that you are not fond of and might hastily dismiss any thought of them. They're changeable. So, see to it you're open to as many new cooking ideas as you can. The seasoning of a sauce, stock, roast, sandwich or many things would be every bit as pleasing with Swiss cheese instead of provolone, ham instead of lamb, black beans instead of hominy, spicy or not…let your taste buds experience new foods.

7— MAIN DISHES SOLO - I'm an unapologetic carnivore. I'm an unapologetic lover of food and don't function well either unsatisfied or hungry. With my life on the line as motivation to rearrange my eating, I was willing to do anything and everything. As you've already seen, I began to look at food, cooking and meals very unlike what's common and it pays off to this very day. Sides and too much variety can over-whelm your good intentions and will power is unreliable, anyway. My meals became more about centered main dishes and sides, breads and dessert (miracle of miracles) all took time off. My nutrition and energy boosts were of the utmost importance while grandiose amounts were out. Veggie troths have been explained, family size salads, too. Many meals have been eggs with no starch or bread sides. 3 eggs scram-bled with veggies - yum, protein power! Chicken means chicken. 4 or 5 pieces with no co-stars from the land of carbs - wow, I'm full yet not stuffed and my level of game is literally multiplied in a matter of minutes. Hot dogs and hamburgers eaten with a knife and fork leave buns in a bag and me getting more meat. 3 or 4 hot dogs dipped in my mustard, relish, onion, hot sauce compote delights and don't keep my pants too tight. Burgers lettuce wrapped or bun-less are bigger. (Grrrrr, I love it. Potatoes may seem like they've been fired here, you couldn't be more wrong. I love spuds. The meat and potato combos have broken up and Mr. Spud is usually a solo star when I have him, too. He is a good guy we've given an undeserved bad reputation to. The glop on it isn't the spud's fault. Steaming hot spuds topped with butter spray (another game changer in the condiment world), onions, veggies (hot OR cold - another use for the unconventional temp twist), beans or meat (protein takes the supporting role, how novel) and you see the light. You can enjoy potatoes not smothered in butter, cheese, sour cream or bacon. You're freeing your mind and the body will fol-low! Now, go enjoy a duck.

8— SCALE PORTIONS BACK - Very tough behavior change for same. This applies to homemade OR bought items. Fattening foods are not eliminated from your life, but the amounts are, to be sure. You must accept this or you'll be struggling on diets that never quite work until your dying day.

Example - celebration cakes come in every size, buy one that covers the amount of expected guests plus two. It's enough. Or make one (see, my non cook mind always switches to buy one, automatically) with the same principle. Don't be afraid to run out. Too many people act as if running out of food will alter the Earth's axis. If you have so many people over and the foods gone, leftover temptations are gone with it! Talk, move away from the table, play a board game, walk it off, have hot tea, take pictures ... live life a new way. When the foods finished, it's probably because everyone's had enough. Dear reader, I'm more concerned about you. Think about the pot of pasta you're making and the amount of people who'll eat it. Transfer this compass to all meals and practice scaling back, then no food is a problem. SOME SNAPPY EXPRESSIONS: It's not the doughnut, it's the dozen. It's not the pizza, it's the pie. It's not the cookie, it's the jar. It's not the fries, it's the super-size. It's not the chocolates, it's the box. It's not the biscuit, it's the basket. Understand, now?

9— RESTAURANTS / PARTIES / FOOD EVENTS SOLVED: Keep it simple. Apples are the secret weapon. Take an apple and eat it in the car on your way to any eat out event. What? Why would I do that? I'm going out to dinner, what good would eating an apple do? SAVE YOU, that's what it'd do. It takes off the edge just enough that you arrive any-place not ravenously starving. This will allow you to behave like a person, not an animal when you arrive. Apples are not written in stone here, they're my fruit of choice because I love them, they travel well (nothing that needs peeled, a plate, knife or fork is a good idea) and a core tossed out as you walk in is easy clean up. Pears can work well. Bananas can work well. Grapes, nectarines.... but apples are best. A big beverage of zero calories next (coffee, tea, diet soda, water...) seals the deal. Go to all social events (family barbeques, business luncheons, showers or any other you may encounter) confident you'll keep your eating managed. You're not too hungry.

10— TEACH KIDS: If these things are what a child sees growing up, it's their normal. They won't have to unlearn too much as an unhappy, unhealthy, overweight adult dealing with damage that they struggle to undo if they don't follow certain paths the adults they love, respect and live with lead them towards. That's one heck of a sentence. It truly can make the difference in an entire generation's destiny. Alas, it needs refocused, too. I know I've provided unconventional ideas here, but they will all work to unlink your addictive food fixation. I never thought I'd be able to feel any relief in my life before I foraged through my tales you're being let into my head for. Now that I'm living life on the other side of the glass, I only want to take the message to overweight people who still suffer and there are millions out there. Are you one of them? If so, I care about you even though I've never met you. I feel for you and believe you'll get success following these loopy directions.

Pass on better food ideas to your kids. Let them live a life with very different hobbies, holiday celebrations, cooking skills and let food take an appropriate place in their lives and not overtake it. Foods commercially mass produced for special occasions only tempt you because of years of conditioning. It can be, <u>must </u>be, unlearned. You wouldn't have bought a marshmallow dipped oval shaped thing at the checkout stand yesterday? Don't buy it because the wrapping paper has a bunny on it. It only makes businessmen richer at your and your kids' expense.

Wise words for all decor, it's just dye! Kids will only get this shot if you allow it. You're that powerful. Use it wisely.

11— KRYPTONITE-LESS HOME: My members get told to remove all fattening foods they're unable to have around them and keep them banned forever, my definition of kryptonite. To this day, I have many foods that are never in my house. I cannot control myself. Yes, after all these years, I'm cured of nothing. I'm at peace about this. I don't expect it to change. That's why all the steps above you happened. Out, we can all enjoy anything. If you live with people who won't allow it, make them feel guilty about this as it's how they should feel. Then, rearrange a pantry, second refrigerator, mini fridge or a negotiated place it will remain. If you think you can leave it there. I know I couldn't, but I'm not you, so you decide. As for kryptonite in the recipe department, is it avoidable? You don't have to repeat previous years of making certain things. The bake sale at church WILL GO ON if you don't make your annual German chocolate cake. It will. You'll be amazed and maybe your ego a bit deflated by how life will not end. A few squawks may occur, but when they're done, you're free. If it's unavoidable, BUY IT ON THE WAY THERE. Don't cook kryptonite. That's like an alcoholic making moonshine, an ex-smoker working in a hookah lounge, a perpetual cheater working in a singles bar. A toxic atmosphere only keeps you on the razor's edge and doesn't bode well for happy endings. I want you to have a happy ending very much.

Well, I'll bet this is unlike any 'recipe' article you've read. To not be modest, I'd match its usefulness against many I've read in a heartbeat. Enjoy!

PROLOGUE TRIPS TO THE STORE:

You have my editor to thank for this section. A comrade in the weight loss battle with some difficulty in the home front reached out to me for a guided tour of a supermarket. He called it revolutionary in his weight loss efforts. How cool is that? I love happy endings and when good things happen to good people.

Some things are always in my house and I highlight them here. Since 'crossing over' I've become fond of the European style of shopping. Meaning I go more often for less things. I find industrial sized refrigerators and freezers overwhelming to me. Who needs to keep that much food on hand? Only large families (lots of kids, not stoutness) could need so much.

When people come over my home, they are quite curious to look in my pantry, icebox (LOVE that old word) and counters. I'm not 100% sure what they're looking for. I can assure you the things I go over in this section are always there. Plus, some carefully selected treats. Yet, I often hear "You have no food in this place!" What?! I have plenty of food. What are you talking about? I have come to a couple of possible translations for this. 1 - My house isn't overflowing in every space with piles of processed food until it resembles the aftermath of a sale at a discount store. Well, ok, I'll grant you that. It doesn't. It never will. 2 - You mean there's no 'junk' in this house. Any home without junk = 'there's nothing to eat'? I see.

Details here are on the basics: The 'can't do withouts'. It's too short, really, much too short. I could have gone on and on. I suppose I have to save some material for book #2. Let me know any helpful thing you use to supplement it. The less you think most people are aware of it, the better.

By the way, to the managers of the many stores who no doubt saw me via surveillance cameras nibbling on open cases of candy and tossing out the wrappers or sampling well beyond what is the unspoken rule of 'just take one, buy any more' that didn't bust me or confront me, I thank you. Did you keep a record of the copious amount of money I spent and let it go? Did you enjoy my pitiful cover up's? Did you feel sorry for me? Were afraid of me? No matter the reason, it's much too late, but, thanks.

X485'S TRIP TO THE STORE:

Grocery stores are not for entertainment. They used to be. As a compulsive overeater in full throttle, going to the store was my version of drinkers going to the bar, compulsive gamblers going to the casino, careless spenders going to the mall. You get the idea. Fun, fun, fun is so many choices and always something new. Now, I shop with purpose and my home remains clean and functional because I'm never without the following things:

Whole rotisserie chickens - Bless whoever brought these to the masses. I have one at all times. Once one is gone, another one comes in. Eaten as snacks by just pulling off a leg, a thigh sliced for a sandwich, microwave the breast and wing to put in soup or have as is — cold, hot, breakfast, lunch, snack, dinner - all made protein packed and they don't cost more than most fast food meals. Indispensable.

Cut up meats - While on the subject, perhaps the most underutilized man in the grocery store - the butcher. Back in the day, the butcher was in the forefront, but has faded and viewed as old fashioned by too many. Processed lunch meats are often full of salt, sugar, preservatives, fat .... all avoidable. Bring the butcher a chicken or turkey breast, a ham, roast beef and tell him to trim the fat and slice it to what size you desire. He says, 'Sure, I'll be back in a few minutes.' He returns with clear wrapped meat in lunch meat manageable portions with unprocessed goodness to be used as healthy, hunger zapping, quick eating all day and all ways.

Fruit, LOTS of it – It shouldn't fit in the traditional fruit drawer. Also, an assignment - buy a new piece of produce every time you're at the store. The off-the-beaten-path is where you'll find a new treat you'll love. You may find things you don't like, but that's how you find diamond treasures. I owe this type of exploration to my discovery of white peaches, all kinds of apples (smitten, ambrosia, jazz, envy), leeks, blood oranges, pearl onions and I know I will find many more as I load up on all that's out there to keep me thin with a grin.

Frozen, quickly re-heatable sauces— This isn't a single item to be bought in a store, but the ingredients you use to make chili, tomato sauce, soups .... it's very useful to take the same amount of time and dishes to wash and eat many times from the effort. Example: grill 12 chicken breasts, wrap 10 of them, put them in the freezer and they're ready. Much faster when you come home tired from work.

Beans - all you like. You know by now I'm a big fan. Carefully selected canned ones are just fine. If you want to soak and blanch, feel free and send same to me!

Full spice rack - Like the produce, you should be able to take a basic dish (chicken, fish, pasta, potatoes, eggs) and make it taste many different ways with the spices you have. Are we going Asian tonight? How about Mexican? Italian? Greek? Spin the globe and you're not eating bland ever again!

Many oils and vinegars - Not in the mood for the same old salad? Me, either. I know how to make a not-the-same-as-yesterday tasting garden grove in a bowl night after night. Makes veggies on the side pop, too.

Ketchup and Mayonnaise packets - Visit your nearest restaurant supply store or just take a whole bunch of them from the condiment stand nearest you. The abuse of gobs of either is virtually eliminated when everyone's squeezing their own individual packets onto their own individual servings. Yes, it's funny at first, but when you lose weight, you'll find most folks are hard pressed to argue with success.

Single portion microwave ready rice - Bless this person, too! Lazy cooking rice lovers of the world thank you! Portion is a problem no more. Ninety seconds and I'm having a perfect portion of white, brown, yellow, Spanish, wild and many other kinds of rice. No pots to clean, will power to stop and carbohydrate itch scratched!

Popsicles - Sugar free, of course. Cold and sweet is a great thing. The fat, calories and potential for abuse in ice cream or novelties is not. I am a major ice cream addict. I find myself incapable of even having the 'diet' kinds around and not abusing. Sigh, I had to bite the bullet and confine myself more than I usually prefer by only keeping these to meet the need for a summer goodie on a stick. Knowing your limitations and not having them in the house = calm, happy thin people.

Popcorn kernels and air popper - Who doesn't like popcorn? I love it, love it. I can't see movies without it, but, gracious, they corrupt it. Only on very indulgent occasions can I go there. Most times, the air popped is fine. Spray it with a margarine spray to give it stick and then apply any dry thing to make it taste like where your mood that night happens to be. Will it be chives, cinnamon, cocoa powder, hot sauce, granulated salt, butter buds? Whichever you choose, comfort food mission complete.

Margarine spray - Bless this one, too! The ability to generally give 'butter' taste to all foods without butter's considerable damage is a gift to the consumer. I spray it on most things and even shot it in my mouth. Thought that habit was just for whipped cream, but time proved me capable of new ideas!

Salsa / Hot sauce - Both indispensable. Hot sauce for heat - I've lived it all my life. Salsa, well, salsa is the new ketchup. You can see the shift in the last 15 years or so. I recall when it was a few brands in a shelf in the Mexican food section. Now, it has rows and many brands. Open up your mind to its uses and BOOM you are adding flavor to your life at all meals and not suffering from the consequences of many dips, dressings and condiments of the past. WORD OF WARNING: as its popularity's grown, there are always companies that'll corrupt it. The days of carte blanche to just about any brand are gone. Look at the label for unwanted things like sugar, corn syrup, fructose, high fat contents, barbeque sauce......

Oatmeal without added sugar - Hot cereal is an old comfort food for many. Now, it, too, has been made as unhealthy as the sugary cereals it used to be compared to so favorably. You, the consumer, must now be on the lookout for the old school stuff. It's still out there in oatmeal, cream of wheat, farina, grits and such, but takes a moment to look for the originals now. Love capitalism, but it does have a seedy underside!

Salad stuff— It should be keeping your veggie drawer full. Splurge on as much as you want with the abandon you used to display when ordering or cooking junk food. Only you know if you'll chop and slice daily and nightly with a good attitude. If you won't, buy the prepared stuff and step into the healthy zone with us. It will be worth lt.

Potatoes - Wrapped, cleaned and ready to heat and eat, I love who's responsible for that being in my stores. The old school hand scrubbed kind are just fine, too. I love potatoes. Most people do. If an unadorned spud without all the old stuff you used to clobber 'em with seems unappealing to you, maybe this is a lesson for you. Do you REALLY like potatoes like you've said you do all these years? Was it just the stuff on top all the time? Try a BITE of a hot potato naked (the spud, not you!) and see what you think. Wow, that's what it tastes like. It's a bit of alright. Now, unhinged from the chains of your past, get creative with your spices and toppings to build perfect snacks or meals with your new friend, the potato.

Salty crackers are the new crouton - I've always liked a bit of crunch on my salad and they provide it. Also, wisely I have them because I like them but don't love them. The brilliance of this compromise has been discussed throughout this book. I don't go crazy on these like a few other brands or types of crackers, so, they're perfect. WORD OF WISDOM: They're great for upset stomachs. They're super absorbent. Believe this.

Individually wrapped cheese slices or sticks - Many people are cheese-o-holics. It's not my top problem food, but I want to help us all. Portion control that is possible to take out of your hands is a golden opportunity every time it's available. Keep realistic about yourself when shopping. Blocks, bowls, slices, bags, shredded and all manors of cheese that's left to your self-control to keep from overdoing is a risk. Don't risk what you can't afford to lose, especially when it's not necessary. WORD OF WISDOM: If you have family (kids, teens, adults) who are reacting to veggie sides with less than the enthusiasm you'd like, put a bit of cheese on the green beans, broccoli, asparagus or mixed medley. The eye appeal of cheese will rope many folks onto your side if they were on the fence. Cheese is good like that!

Light breads, English muffins, tortillas - Healthy eating must be more profitable than I thought. Hooray! There are bread items that are more weight control friendly all over now. Admittedly, I'm not a bread-o-holic, but I still say this - It's not meant to be special bread. It's just a dry vessel to transport the contents of a sandwich, breakfast, burrito, quesadilla.... into your mouth. Seen thus, it doesn't have to be special. Save that for when it's on its own and you're focused on it exclusively. That's for the dinner roll or deli style and the happiness it'll provide when it's savored. But for regular day to day lunches and such, please consider the light breads. You're wise to.

Eggs - Useful for much more than breakfast. I have always liked traditionally breakfast type foods for lunch or dinner, as well. Also, hard boiled eggs are awesome protein pick-ups you can have at work very easily. Top salads and such.... you know that already. Did you know they're available in twos PEELED? Woo Hoo, who's with me at the party celebrating another victory for the non- cook? Woot Woot!

Broth - Ready to use makes for moist meats, soups, bases for stews and to assist if your meat was so low fat, it's a bit dry. Cheap and versatile and with next to no calories, It's a tool for eating well.

Shrimp - There isn't a bad one on the planet, it seems. This healthy and super tasting creature deserves applause for how satisfying it is.

Hot or cold, breakfast, lunch or dinner, baby size to colossal, fancy to picnic, kid to adult, it's rare to find such an across the board pleaser like him. Learn many ways to season him. He takes very well to multiple kinds of vinegars, to start.

TV dinners —I call them this word intentionally due to its outdated-ness. Frozen meals, if you please, have come a very long way. Being in the diet game since I was 9 or so, I can vouch for this. The 'diet' ones used to taste terrible. Not so, anymore. The choices are many and the places they can help you out, too. Have them at work. You can't always predict how you'll feel next week. The frozen meal is waiting for your last minute decision that lunch out or down the hall at the cafeteria isn't a good idea. If you're on vacation and have a mini fridge / freezer and a microwave, you save a fortune on room service. At home, they're the new wise person's snacks. This is discussed in the book many places, too. Use them very strategically. Not enough for a meal, perhaps, but, as snacks, perfect. WORD OF WISDOM: Have no inhibitions about having them in the morning if you're vulnerable to the unhealthy options in your world when hunger rears its head late in the morning or mid-afternoon.

Well, if you have a grocery trip like this, you're moving in the right direction. Learn when your store gives out samples and DON'T GO THEN. Also, don't go hungry. It's asking for disaster. In fact, a good game plan here - go right after a meal - when it's the last thing you want to do. You'd be amazed how unpleasant being around all that food is when you're full. "NO, I don't want a taste of that" and "Stick to the list" may come out of your mouth unforced. You might go home in wonder, thinking, 'I've never done the family shopping quicker in my life.' or 'I didn't spend a penny on a single impulse item. That's amazing!' Shopping on a full tummy makes it happen.

INVITATION TO RESPOND:

What did you think? I hope you found it worth your time. I thank you for allowing me to bring you into the fold for this glimpse of what can happen when you take the brave step to take your approach to food on and make the lifestyle change you've read so much of by now.

I hear you breathe heavily in public, I feel for your pain, I see you struggle in the heat getting your day to day tasks done, I smell the foods that are everywhere that tempt us and I say how fixable this is to some of you. I know you even though we will never meet. Your clothes either don't fit or are elastic. You're taking meds to manage your life you'd likely not need if you lost weight. I see you in buffets eating so much. I see you in the discount stores stocking up on cheap eats. I've been you in all those situations.

I see you try valiantly to improve this over and over. If you've allowed previous disappointments to lure you into giving up, consider this book a wake up alarm. You don't have to live like that anymore. Even if your friends are all overweight, you've begun to accept rationalizations to remain heavy, simply avoid mirrors and follow bogus trends on the hope that the miracles offered may work. You may have identified with some stories like I'd had surveillance cameras on you. I promise I didn't. Some stories are completely unlike your own life, but you read them to see what happens to them. If this is true, it's likely you have the courage and determination to become a slim healthy person, too.

I am quite eager to hear your opinion of this book. My invitation to respond covers any sections that spoke to you. What was most helpful, funny, close to home sounds hard to believe, difficult to understand, food tricks you're surprised were so good, disagreeable suggestions that you'd like to counter offer better. I want to improve and I need feedback for this. My desire to connect to a wider audience is only beginning. There is a new book in the works and I'll want even more input from the public for it. I can't tell you the title yet, because it's not definite, but it's good. More on book #2 as it develops.

For now, in conclusion, if you learned something in this book that has motivated you to get your weight under control, then I've accomplished my primary goal. If you learned more than a small bit, I'm over the moon glad for you. Keep in touch. Send me your success stories, progressions, frustrations, surprise foods you discover.... whatever is working, so it can be passed on to anyone with a computer.

Wake up call delivered. I'm reaching out my hand. The next move is yours. You can do this!